Praise for The Thought Propels the Sound *from voice trainers . . .*

". . . *The Thought Propels the Sound* will fill a vacuum in the field of performance literature. Although there are many books available to actors on how to train their voices—and actors know that they must train their voices—there is an astonishing level of—let's call it —deafness in directors, artistic directors, and producers. This book promises to sound a necessary alarm that will penetrate to those who wield authority over actors and very often jeopardize a performance because their eyes dominate their creative process. In simple terms, the information Feindel offers will sensitize directors, empower actors, and guide vocal coaches, trainers, and speech pathologists. The book is practical and opens up a subject that has too long remained somewhat mysterious to the non-initiate. Voices need to be talked about. In particular, directors need to know how the voice works and how to maximize the conditions for the most vivid and appropriate vocal life on stage. It is interesting that in training programs for directors there are courses in lighting, scene design, and script analysis, but not in voice. And yet voice and language are the heartbeat of Western theater. Certainly in England a voice teacher/coach/text-director is almost always part of the creative team that is assembled for a production. The National Theatre and the Royal Shakespeare Company have one or more voice directors on staff. In the States this concept has yet to be generally accepted. Perhaps because the role of auteur-director is preeminent, or perhaps because the contribution of a voice director has not been understood. Janet Feindel's book will go a long way to dispel misunderstanding, educate, and illuminate the art that is speaking."

—Kristin Linklater, Professor of Voice and Head of Acting, Theatre Division, Columbia University, author of *Freeing the Natural Voice* and *Freeing Shakespeare's Voice*

"Janet has the expertise and commitment to quality that I prize when working with master teachers and voice and speech coaches. She has a unique ability to add a fresh perspective to a director who may not be familiar with the principles of vocal work, while at the same time honoring the vocal health of the actors."

—Paul Wagar, Artistic Director, Ark Theatre Company, Los Angeles; Voice/Speech Faculty, MFA Acting Program, School of Theater, Film, and Television, UCLA

. . . from Alexander teachers:

"Janet Madelle Feindel brings a unique perspective to acting voice in that she combines her in-depth knowledge of various established modalities of voice, including the work of Kristin Linklater, with her expertise as an Alexander teacher, gearing her insights for directors and anyone interested in the actor's voice. She constantly pursues new ideas and ways to refine her already-proven methods. She has worked with top professionals in the field and brings a fresh and much-needed approach to this area with wit, intelligence, and a wealth of experience."

—Michael D. Frederick, Director, Alexander Technique Workshops-International and founding director of the first three International Congresses on the F. M. Alexander Technique

. . . from directors, artistic directors, producers, and playwrights:

"Finally—a book from Janet Feindel. This is a voice teacher in demand for a good reason: her students are consistently at the forefront of the acting profession. One of a handful of supreme vocal coaches in the English-speaking world, Janet is unique in that she is a Designated Linklater voice teacher, also certified in Fitzmaurice *and* Alexander. Her ability to incorporate this physical work with the voice training has put her into a category all her own. We will absorb her insights about thought-linked voice with eager pleasure."

> —Martha Henry, Officer of the Order of Canada, recipient of the Governor General's Lifetime Achievement Award in the Performing Arts, Order of Ontario, actress, director, former artistic director, Director of the Birmingham Conservatory, Stratford Shakespeare Festival

"This is a much-needed text. Why didn't someone think of this sooner?"

> —The late Milan Stitt, playwright (*Runner Stumbles*, *Hunting Accidents*), screenwriter (*Long Shadows*), Raymond Smith Professor of Dramatic Writing, School of Drama, Carnegie Mellon University, and former Executive Director of Circle Repertory Theater

"It has been my pleasure to work with Janet Feindel on a number of productions over 15 years and I have witnessed firsthand the impact of her coaching.

"Janet has worked with many of the world's top directors and has a strong sense of what aspects of voice and Alexander work will enhance a director's approach through rehearsal and into the run. This kind of skillful support for a director's vision can make a vital difference to the quality of a production.

"Janet's talent and her ability to fuse a number of different methods make her contribution unique."

> —Antoni Cimolino, Director General, Stratford Shakespeare Festival, Canada

"Janet Feindel zeroes in on a vitally important and often overlooked area: how the director supports the actors' work on text and voice. Her new book, *The Thought Propels the Sound*, is a refreshing and illuminating guide for directors, artistic directors, actors, and vocal coaches."

> —Jeffrey Horowitz, Artistic Director, Theatre for a New Audience, New York City

"I have been directing movies and television for over 20 years and I have always found the soul of an actor's performance to live in the sound of his or her voice. I have found Janet Feindel's insights into an actor's physical and emotional preparation through voice to be inspired. *The Thought Propels the Sound* is a must-read for any director."

> —Graeme Campbell, director, including *Murder One*, *Old Fashioned Thanksgiving* and *Everest*, and recipient, Gemini award for *You Can't Always Get What You Want*

"This is a significant book that pays attention to an important area for directors. I know Janet Madelle Feindel's excellent work firsthand and her book makes a distinctive and welcome contribution, creating a new paradigm."

> —Mladen Kiselov, director, Professor Emeritus, former head of directing, Carnegie Mellon University School of Drama

"As a performing arts center manager for almost two decades, I welcome this unique addition to the literature of the field. Every arts presenter should have this volume on their shelf, and recognize that the advice it contains could make the difference between a successful engagement or a possible artist cancellation. As a regular public speaker, I use my voice frequently as a representative of my arts organization, and I have been the fortunate beneficiary of Janet Feindel's accessible and easily understood teaching."

> —Janice Price, C.E.O., Luminato, Toronto Festival of the Arts and Creativity; former C.E.O., Kimmel Center for Performing Arts, Philadelphia

... from actors:

"Janet Madelle Feindel has a plethora of attributes, but for the sake of economy, let me list two: (1) I (and my colleagues at CMU, where we took her class) still use Madelle's exercises in our professional careers, as they are practical, simple, and extremely beneficial, and

(2) unlike [that of] other voice teachers, Madelle's work helps an actor support one's choices with proper vocal support, as opposed to limiting one's choices with some stodgy idea of what 'the voice' should sound like in a theatrical context."

> —Christopher Hoch, Broadway roles include Tony Parker in *Die Mommy Die*, Sir Lancelot in *Spamalot*, and Gaston in *Beauty and the Beast* (Broadway and national tour), and appearances on *30 Rock*

... from voice scientists:

"Since the late 1970s, an extraordinary volume of scientific and medical information has been amassed and applied to voice medicine, science, therapy, training, and performance. Physicians, speech-language pathologists, and singing teachers recognized the value of this new information and interdisciplinary collaboration immediately, and began applying it for the benefit of their patients and students. Soon, voice and speech trainers joined the interdisciplinary effort. Pioneers such as Bonnie Raphael, Cicely Berry, Patsy Rodenburg, Kristin Linklater, Catherine Fitzmaurice, and others became involved early. Their knowledge helped healthcare providers understand vocal injury and professional voice demands, as well as improve therapy for actors and other professional speakers. The knowledge they acquired through interaction with other disciplines enhanced their understanding of the voice and increased the sophistication of their analysis and understanding of actors' voices. Such knowledge also helped their intervention techniques evolve. In about 1995, Sharon L. Freed became the first voice trainer to be employed in a physician's office and part of a medical voice team, creating a paradigm through which voice trainers could help enhance vocal health and performance.

"Through her association with the Voice Foundation and her academic and theatrical activities, Janet Feindel has been involved intimately with the evolution of this field for many years. Her book synthesizing pertinent knowledge and reducing it to the information most practical for directors is excellent, and overdue. It should be of great value in helping directors and voice trainers enhance the health and endurance of their actors' voices while enhancing their ability to express artistic emotion. Hopefully, it will also help decrease the number of vocal injuries that lead professionals to require laryngologic care. The information in this book provides an invaluable introduction to the state of the art, and it should be read by anyone involved in voice training."

> —Robert T. Sataloff, MD, DMA,
> Chairman of the American Voice Foundation

... *from theater educators and practitioners:*

"Janet Feindel has developed an expert, yet personal approach to the important business of training the actor's voice. Hers is one which takes into account the varied challenges that the current generation of actors and directors will encounter as they are called upon to engage with how theater will be defined in the 21st century. It should be considered an essential complement to established resources in the field."

> —Elizabeth Bradley, Chair of NYU's undergraduate School of Drama; Cultural Ambassador for the Stratford Shakespeare Festival; Producer, Festival of Firsts; and former Head of Drama at Carnegie Mellon University

"Contemporary theater, reflecting as it does a fast-moving, impatient world, all too often ignores the power of live speech, of the words spoken with deliberation and conviction. Janet Madelle Feindel's book is an invaluable aid to the work of the theater director in this crucial area. Combining personal insight with a solid technical basis, Ms. Feindel brings to bear decades of practical experience gained while teaching and coaching at the highest levels of our profession."

> —Dr. Vladimir Mirodan, Principal,
> Drama Center, London, UK

"I have had the pleasure of working (as both an actor and director) with Janet Madelle Feindel as a vocal coach and found her to be incredibly knowledgeable, vital, and effective. Now, with her wonderful book, *The Thought Propels the Sound*, everyone can benefit from Janet's enormous knowledge and vitality! And, if everyone incorporates Janet's techniques, they will find it as effective as I did working with her. I highly recommend this book to anyone remotely interested in the actors' process. For directors, it is a must-read!"

> —John Shepard, actor, director, author of
> *Auditioning and Acting for the Camera*,
> and Chair of the Theatre Department at
> Point Park University

The Thought
Propels the Sound

The Thought Propels the Sound

Janet Madelle Feindel, MFA

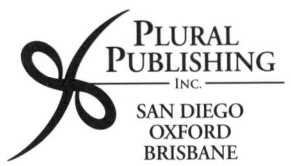

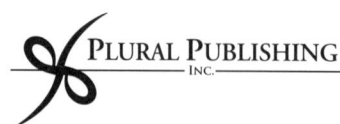

5521 Ruffin Road
San Diego, CA 92123

e-mail: info@pluralpublishing.com
Web site: http://www.pluralpublishing.com

49 Bath Street
Abingdon, Oxfordshire OX14 1EA
United Kingdom

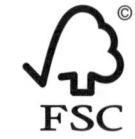

FSC
Mixed Sources
Product group from well-managed
forests and other controlled sources

Cert no. SW-COC-002283
www.fsc.org
© 1996 Forest Stewardship Council

Copyright © by Plural Publishing, Inc. 2009

Typeset in 11/13 Garamond by Flanagan's Publishing Services, Inc.
Printed in the United States of America by McNaughton and Gunn, Inc.

Cover photo of Janet Madelle Feindel working with Eric Berryman (BFA, Acting student, School of Drama, Carnegie Mellon University) and author photo by Karen Waggoner.

All rights, including that of translation, reserved. No part of this publication may be reproduced, stored in a retrieval system, or transmitted in any form or by any means, electronic, mechanical, recording, or otherwise, including photocopying, recording, taping, Web distribution, or information storage and retrieval systems without the prior written consent of the publisher.

For permission to use material from this text, contact us by
Telephone: (866) 758-7251
Fax: (888) 758-7255
e-mail: permissions@pluralpublishing.com

To inquire about translation and media rights, contact the author's agent, Susan Schulman, at Susan Schulman Literary Agency, 454 West 44th St., New York, NY 10036, USA, or Schulman@aol.com.

Every attempt has been made to contact the copyright holders for material originally printed in another source. If any have been inadvertently overlooked, the publishers will gladly make the necessary arrangements at the first opportunity.

Library of Congress Cataloging-in-Publication Data

Feindel, Janet M.
  The thought propels the sound / Janet M. Feindel.
    p. cm.
  Includes bibliographical references and index.
  ISBN-13: 978-1-59756-206-5 (alk. paper)
  ISBN-10: 1-59756-206-8 (alk. paper)
  1. Voice culture. 2. Voice. I. Title.
  PN4162.F38 2009
  808.5—dc22

2009004341

Contents

Preface	xv
Acknowledgments	xxii
Contributors	xxiv

1	Introduction to Voice Training	1
2	Overview of Voice Methods: Whose Voice Is It Anyway?	13
3	Overview of Speech Methods: Whose Standard Is It Anyway?	31
4	Voice and the Alexander Technique	45
5	Vox Explora: What Is It?	61
6	Resonex	87
7	Voice and Text Explorations	111
8	Directors, Voice, and the Rehearsal Process	133
9	Special Issues	149
10	Working with Voice/Dialect and Alexander Coaches	165

References	191
Resources	193
Appendix: Anatomy and Physiology of the Voice	211
Index	245

Preface

As a young actress, I had the good fortune to work at the Stratford Shakespeare Festival under the artistic directorship of Robin Phillips. Instinctively, I knew that this was a unique opportunity as I was able to observe the work of some of the world's most gifted actors: Brian Bedford, Brent Carver, Patricia Conolly, Martha Henry, Marti Maraden, Richard Monette, Maggie Smith, Jessica Tandy, and Peter Ustinov, along with many others. Over the years, I have become increasingly aware of how this experience shaped my sensibility both as an actor and as a coach.

During that time, I was in a production of *Love's Labor's Lost*, directed by Robin Phillips, in which Martha Henry[1] played the Princess of France. I listened to Henry speak these lines for several months.[2] Her voice embodied the vulnerability of every moment, particularly at the point where the princess is informed of the death of her father. To this day, when I hear this text spoken, I still hear the nuances of Henry's voice, as the memory of her delicate sound remains indelibly imprinted in my brain. It is more than just how her voice "sounded," though surely she has a most beautiful voice. More importantly, it was what her voice evoked, and how the vibrations of her voice conveyed the inner life of the character, revealing the joy and sadness along with a multitude of other textures of each moment in this character's life. The sound had also to be incredibly powerful, given the fact that she effortlessly filled the 1800 or so seats in the Stratford Festival Theatre, with absolute ease.

---

[1] Martha Henry is a Companion of the Order of Canada and a member of the Order of Ontario and has received the Governor General's Lifetime Achievement Award in the Performing Arts. She has received seven honorary doctorates, five Genie Awards, three Gemini Awards, and two Sterling Awards. An actress and director, she is presently director of the Birmingham Conservatory for Classical Theatre at the Stratford Shakespeare Festival of Canada.

[2] Often, the Stratford shows in the long season go from May until as late as November.

As a voice/Alexander and dialect teacher and coach, I know that striking this delicate balance is the ongoing challenge.

Over the years, I have worked with many directors who I assume want what Martha Henry achieved, whether they articulate this or not. Sometimes, however, the director does not know how to help an actor find this balance or how to help the actor maintain it through the course of rehearsal and performance. I wrote this book in the hope that directors and those studying to become directors will take the time to learn about the voice, so they have at least an inkling of its delicate interplay of the actor's process and the actor's voice and how these two processes are intrinsically linked. How can directors develop in such a way that they stimulate and nurture the most expressive and delicate release of nuance through the voice in a way that can touch an audience deeply and leave a lasting visceral impression on an audience?

There are, of course, many practical reasons for directors to understand the voice. When an actor loses his or her voice, it creates many problems in a rehearsal or performance schedule. Putting on an understudy is a costly and stressful venture. When audiences complain about lack of audibility or clarity, this is clearly not helpful to the success of a production. Most theater directors understand that one wants to hear and understand an actor clearly. Most can see why it would not be practical to have actors straining their voices and going hoarse on a continuous basis with eight shows a week for an extended time. What is a director to do when an actor loses his voice? If actors and singers are expected to perform unhealthy vocal tasks on a regular basis, the performer often suffers the consequences for many years to come (although some producers seem not to concern themselves with this fact).

On a deeper level, however, there are tools that will help directors stimulate and nurture the actor's voice so that it can reveal the inner soul of the character and still be strong and clear enough to be heard and be sustained over a long theatrical run or many hours of a film shoot, where a director may need to reshoot an intense scene many times. The training of the voice involves many complex areas. There are the mechanics, the anatomy and health of the voice, and the deeper, less explicable aspects that involve the emotion, the spirit, the psychology of the individual, and the political and sociological influences of a given culture.

If the voice reveals the spirit of the character in a manner that is deeply connected to the character and the actor's psyche and interior life, with the voice vibrations freely releasing through the whole body, the audience experiences the play in a deep, instinctive way. They may not surmise that it is the voice connection that makes the difference between an experience of theater that's "Yeah, that was okay" and a piece of theater that moves us to the core. They may only realize that there's a difference between something mildly satisfying and something deeply affecting. Since voice is about the delicate interplay of breath, the momentum of thought, kinesthetic experience, and personalization of words and images, it is the springboard from which the rest of the play stems. If an actor can't connect the breath and the sound, how can she communicate a whole play for 3 hours in any kind of authentic, revealing way?

It is possible to use the voice as a mask. If one concerns oneself with "sounding" good, rather than concerning oneself with what one is communicating, the delivery becomes affected, and this never fully satisfies an audience. A voice connected to the deep need of the character always sounds good no matter what, because it grows out of the soul of the character and draws the audience in.

WHY DIRECTORS NEED VOICE TRAINING

A director sets the tone of a production, while an artistic director sets the tone of a theater; however, both director and artistic director have the opportunity to encourage healthy and expressive voice usage. The free voice, integrated with the actor's intention and fully connected with the actor's body, will affect the audience at a deeper level, creating a more exciting artistic experience.

Over the last 30 years there have been great strides in voice training in a number of areas. The status of the voice or speech coach has changed, and voice and speech training has become much more sophisticated. Many methods exist, and voice and speech training has incorporated principles and approaches from a number of other fields including yoga, Feldenkrais, Alexander Technique, bioenergetics, voice science, and psychology. Voice science has become a recognized field of study.

There are clinics devoted to interdisciplinary approaches to voice care all over the world. The Voice Foundation, under the leadership of Robert Sataloff, MD, DMA, based in Philadelphia, sponsors the annual Care of the Professional Voice Symposium, an interdisciplinary conference dealing with all aspects of voice care: voice anatomy, acoustics, singing and speaking voice training, treatment and surgery for voice disorders, interdisciplinary voice teams, and injury prevention. Twenty years ago, it was the only interdisciplinary conference of its kind, but now many such international voice symposiums meet on a regular basis. The Voice Foundation also sponsored the first interdisciplinary clinic devoted to the care of the professional voice, in which a team of otolaryngologists, speech pathologists, singing teachers, as well as voice and speech teachers collaborates to give the professional voice user the best treatment possible. Today such clinics exist all over the world.

The Voice and Speech Trainers Association (VASTA), which started as a tiny organization, now has hundreds of members. VASTA sponsors workshops, conferences, the *Voice and Speech Review*, a newsletter, and a Web site. Voice and speech training has become recognized as a legitimate field. A number of voice and speech professionals hold prestigious positions. Kristin Linklater, author of *Freeing the Natural Voice* and a great pioneer in voice training in the United States, is a professor at Columbia University. Dr. Dudley Knight, one of the leading teachers of the Fitzmaurice method and an innovator in speech training, is vice-chair emeritus of the Irvine Drama Program at the University of California. Even small liberal arts theater programs generally include voice and speech training in their acting curriculum.

Directors are expected to understand theater history, aspects of design, and stage management, but rarely do they receive any training in basic voice and speech or even text analysis. They know that the speaking voice is important, but often they do not know how to communicate or reinforce principles of healthy voice usage. With the best of intentions, they frequently give suggestions to actors that actually encourage vocal tension. This is true even of many talented and established directors. A recent issue of *American Theatre Magazine*[3] included an article on training directors with not a word

---

[3] "Panel on Directing, Moderated by Michael Bloom, with Liz Diamond, Jon Jory, Hal Scott, and Mel Shapiro," *American Theatre Magazine*, January 2002, p. 26.

on voice and speech training as part of a director's preparation. We might assume that the principles of healthy voice usage would be common knowledge and an obvious concern. This, unfortunately, is seldom the case.

TITLES AND CREDIT

In the sports world, a coach is a person of high status, but with voice and speech coaches, the opposite is true. Even relatively high-status coaches working on films do not receive "star" billing or anything close to it. Their names usually appear late in the list of credits. In theater, voice or speech coaches can often negotiate front page billing with the director and designers, but some companies still bury coaching credits in the back of the program, thus misrepresenting the coach's contribution. The voice/text person contributes greatly to the overall success of the production and can enhance the work of a director immeasurably.

The title of a voice and speech trainer has not been clearly defined. They may use *voice and speech coach*, *voice and speech director*, or *voice and speech consultant*. The title can reflect the extent of the voice and speech trainer's input, or represent the sensibility of the community with which the voice and speech trainer is working. The business community, for example, generally uses the word *consultant*. Coaches working on film productions sometimes list themselves as *dialogue coach* or *dialect consultant*. In part, this confusion about appropriate titles reflects the fact that the field of voice and speech training is in the process of defining itself. People often think speaking voice coaches are singing coaches. The title *speech coach* can also be misleading. In the United States at least, a speech coach is someone who teaches speech sounds, pronunciation, and dialects. Training in voice production deals with breath support, resonance, range, text analysis, and ways for actors to integrate the principles of healthy voice usage. Not every speech coach necessarily deals with voice production and visa versa.

Many coaches also incorporate text analysis into their work and may, therefore, use the title *voice/text coach, voice/text director*, or, depending on the time commitment, *voice/text consultant*. If the coach's responsibility includes dialects and accents, the coach should be called *voice and dialect coach*, *voice and dialect director*, or simply *dialect consultant*. In my own case, I am trained as an Alexander teacher and this impacts all aspects of my approach to my work, so where possible I like to include that in my title: "voice/dialect/Alexander coach" or "voice/text/Alexander consultant (or director)." If a coach is working on a musical, it is helpful to indicate that the coach deals with clarity of lyrics and speech in order to differentiate his role from that of the singing vocal coach or musical director. For example, in this instance, "voice/speech/text consultant," "voice/speech/text coach," or "voice/speech/text director" works well. The main point is that the contribution of the voice person, which may also include text, dialect, and occasionally the Alexander Technique, should be recognized appropriately on the first page in the theater program, along with the director, designer, stage manager, and so on, and their bio included in the program.

In Shakespeare's *Romeo and Juliet*, Juliet asks, "What's in a name?" Surely a coach's work should be more important than his title—but not necessarily. For a profession that is in the process of defining itself, titles are important. Voice coaches need to be assertive. They must insist on being included in the collaborative process of a production as vital participants rather than as "servants." The problem may be partly due to the fact that the field has tended to attract more women than men. The actual task of defining the voice and speech coach's title is challenging. According to many feminists, women traditionally shy away from seeking credit, but it is important that all coaches, male or female, receive appropriate recognition. It is important that directors support coaches in this endeavor, treating them as collaborators, just as they do costume and set designers.

The study of voice and speech from a director's perspective should be an integral aspect of training for directors. They should understand basic principles of voice and speech production, ways to integrate voice and speech principles with text analysis, methods for working effectively with voice coaches, and strategies for preventing vocal injury. Directors should develop a foundation in voice and speech just as they develop a foundation in other aspects of a production, such as staging, design, theater history, and stage management. Directing courses in liberal arts and conservatory programs should include voice and speech as part of the core training.

My hope is that in reading this book, directors will commit to the importance of voice in the theater at every level; that directors will guide actors to use the words as their gifts and weapons, allowing the thought to propel the sound, with a strong kinesthetic and heartfelt relationship to language so actors can move audiences to the core of their being; that directors and artistic directors will more appropriately recognize and utilize the contribution of voice, text, and Alexander coaches and value their contribution in the same manner they do the creative contributions of designers and other members of the artistic team. By providing directors with basic education in voice, speech, and text, we can increase the possibility of dynamic theater that truly speaks to us.

Janet Madelle Feindel

Acknowledgments

This journey of finding my voice has proven much more exciting than I could have ever imagined and, like in most things, I did not travel it alone.

Thank you to the Tyrone Guthrie Committee at the Stratford Shakespeare Festival, Kent State University Research and Sponsored Programs, the Berkman Faculty Development Fund, and the College of Fine Arts, Carnegie Mellon University. Special thanks to Dr. Susan Ambrose, associate provost and director of the Eberly Center for Teaching Excellence, Carnegie Mellon University, for all her guidance in helping me develop Resonex and for her ongoing support; my agent, Susan Schulman, for her belief in my talent; my dear colleague, Martin Prekop, former dean of the College of Fine Arts, Carnegie Mellon, for all his mentoring; Barbara Anderson, associate dean of the College of Fine Arts, Carnegie Mellon; Dr. Hilary Robinson, dean of the College of Fine Arts, Carnegie Mellon; Dr. Indira Nair, Vice Provost for Education, Carnegie Mellon; and Dr. Mark Kamlet, Provost, Carnegie Mellon.

Thank you to the staff of Plural Publishing for their commitment to voice care.

A special expression of gratitude to David Smukler, Head of Voice, York University, for his generous guidance. Thanks, thanks, and ever thanks to Cicely Berry, OBE, Director of Voice, Royal Shakespeare Company; Lucinda Holshue, Vocal Coach, Guthrie Theater/University of Minnesota Theatre program; Kristin Linklater, Professor, Columbia University; and Robert Sataloff, MD, DMA, Chair of the Voice Foundation, for their support on the book. Thank you to Catherine Fitzmaurice, Lynne Innerst, Dudley Knight, Joan Melton, Tom Murray, Katherine Verdolini, Andrew Wade, Paul Wagar, and Kate Wilson.

Also thank you to my colleagues at Carnegie Mellon University's School of Drama: Cathy Morrow, Mladen Kiselov, Peter Frisch, Elizabeth Bradley, Gregory Lehane, Don Marinelli, Cindy Limauro, Keith

Marsh, and Gina Kuhn. For giving me the encouragement to embark on the Alexander teacher training, I thank Ingrid Sonnichsen, Barbara Mackenzie-Wood, Anthony McKay, and Don Wadsworth. Thank you to the inspiring Alexander Technique community, including Karin Boskins (and the German Alexander Alliance teachers), Bruce Fertman, Michael Frederick, Zoana Gebner-Mueller, Martha Hansen-Fertman, Carolyn Johnston, Pamela Lewis, Frank Ottiwell, Judy Stern, Elizabeth Walker, Lucia Walker, and Anne Waxman. Thank you also to my former colleagues at Kent State University: Drs. Rosemarie K. Bank, Marya Bednerik, Barry Daniels, Richard Klick, and Peter Mueller.

Thank you to Martha Henry, OC, Antoni Cimolino (General Director of the Stratford Shakespeare Festival) and the late Richard Monette, former artistic director, and the late Michael Mawson, former director of the conservatory (who inspired the title of this book).

Thank you to my husband, Robert Haley, for his unending patience and help through this process, my parents, William Feindel, OC, MDCM, and Faith Feindel, RN, my family, Judy Redpath, and Billy Sutherland for their encouragement and love.

Thanks to Deborah Clipperton, Robin Connors, Paula Hill, Louise Penny, Karen Schulze, and Karen Waggoner.

I am grateful to the wonderful actors and directors I have worked with and, of course, my talented, dynamic, "fabulous and flexible" acting students in Carnegie Mellon's School of Drama and the University of California at Los Angeles' Department of Theater, Film, and Television.

And finally, a huge thank you to Lisa Ritter for her invaluable editorial help and moral support—I simply could not have done this without her.

Contributors

Katherine Verdolini Abbott, PhD, CCC-SLP
Professor
Communication Sciences and Disorders
School of Health and Rehabilitation Sciences
University of Pittsburgh
Pittsburgh, Pennsylvania
Appendix

Aaron Ziegler, BA, BFA, MA
University of Pittsburgh
Pittsburgh, Pennsylvania
Appendix

CHAPTER 1

Introduction to Voice Training

We listen to the actor because the thought propels the story forward. Often, the most effective voice usage goes unnoticed because we become concerned with character, plot, and relationships—which is as it should be. In general, people only notice the voice usage when it impedes the listener's ability to become fully involved with the story.

Many young actors initially have difficulty understanding the need for voice training. "I talk already, right?" The example I give is this: I may well run to the bus stop but that does not mean I can run in the Olympics. Most people speak; actors, however, require Olympic vocal ability. They need to develop vocal range, flexibility, and expressiveness in order to maintain vocal freedom under varying degrees of stressful circumstances.

A usual run for actors in the theater involves an average of 8 shows a week, sometimes as many as 10. Even the promise of overtime pay does not make up for potential vocal difficulties. Actors working on a film may need to endure long shoots starting in the early morning or going late into the night. These situations all have the potential to create vocal strain for the actor. The director can be of enormous support to actors in maintaining healthy voice use.

There may be financial implications of poor voice usage as well. Because the majority of theater engagements tend not to be high paying, many actors need to work at other things at the same time, such as reading for book DVDs, voice-over, animation, and so on, so it is important that they keep their voices healthy. Actors may enjoy successful careers in voice-over and animation, but if they don't know how to properly use and take care of their voices, they can lose this valuable source of income.

WHAT IS HEALTHY, EXPRESSIVE, EFFECTIVE VOICE USAGE?

Because many actors or directors may not have given much thought to voice usage, it may be useful to consider in more detail what good voice usage entails.

Describing voice usage is challenging. In the realm of speech pathology and acoustics, we measure breath capacity and fundamental frequencies. This does not, however, give us much information about what we need to know in artistic terms. Voice usage works effectively when we easily hear what the actor is saying; we understand easily what the actor is saying; and, most importantly, we care about what the actor is saying.

Good voice usage is healthy. By this I mean that the sound is full and unencumbered, with no raspiness. The tone is clear. The voice carries effortlessly, filling a large space. The actor uses proper breath support and does not tighten in the throat area. The audience can relax as they are listening to the actor speak.

Good voice usage is expressive. The actor communicates the nuances of the text to the audience through inflection, use of range and vocal dynamics, phrasing, and an overall sense of musicality of the language. Most importantly, the actor's voice stems from the impulse of the thought. It seems easy and spontaneous to the listener. The actor embodies the muscularity of the language and the inherent rhythm and onomatopoeia of the words. The voice reveals the inner yearnings of the character through the text as well as the ideas.

Good voice usage is effective. The diction expresses the thoughts clearly; the audience can comfortably understand what is being said without the actor enunciating in an unnatural manner. We as the audience are not aware of the actor's diction but of the clarity of the actor's thoughts. If a dialect is used, it should not overshadow the rest of the performance but blend into the overall characterization.

WHAT CONSTITUTES POOR VOICE USAGE?

Poor voice usage is unhealthy. Vocal misuse can lead to various vocal difficulties such as inflammation or vocal nodules. These sorts of vocal problems can lead to loss of range, and hoarseness. These symptoms are sometimes temporary and treatable and in other instances lead to long-term vocal damage. We can identify unhealthy voice use in a number of ways. The actor's voice sounds hoarse, thin, and uneven in tone. The voice breaks when changing register so much so that it distracts from the meaning. It is difficult to decipher what is being said and sometimes to hear what is being said at all. The voice usage is monotone. It feels "pushed" and strident. As an audience, we seem to sense the actor's tension in our own bodies. At the other end of the spectrum, the voice sounds breathy, disconnected, and has a disembodied quality to it, what we refer to as *off voice*. The only way to know absolutely if there is actual vocal fold damage is for a doctor to examine the vocal folds through laryngoscopy. (See Appendix.)

Poor voice is inexpressive. The actor's pitch range is limited. There is little resonance. The voice does not convey the nuance of the text. The actor's voice usage does not honor the musicality of the language. It is one note, lacking in dynamics and inflection.

Poor voice usage is ineffective. The voice does not communicate the plot of the play or film. The actor's lack of breath support and tension interferes with the audience's ability to perceive what is being said. This can happen in a passionate scene where the actor's emotions can easily eclipse the intellectual substance of the scene. One must always look for appropriate balance here.

Many voices can communicate relatively undemanding text but the true test comes when an actor must deal with material involving higher intensity, such as the work of Shakespeare or an intense emotional scene in a film. It takes years of training and expertise to maintain breath support and clarity with a sense of authenticity under these circumstances.

Controversial Voice Usage

Controversial voice usage is effective on one level in that the voice is true to the character demands of the play or script, but it employs a vocal quality that could be damaging over a period of time. The trick here is to find a way to create the illusion of the desired quality without vocal misuse. Resonex, as outlined in Chapter 6, can prove useful here. Resonex explores ways of developing awareness of resonating areas while maintaining proper breath support. This encourages actors to discover ways to make vocal choices that do not put undue strain on the vocal apparatus. When actors experiment with vocal qualities, often their first instinct is to produce the sound by tightening in the throat. This tends to be true in dialect use as well. Exploring resonating areas, with full support, gives the actor and director a healthy way to experiment with various vocal qualities and placements for dialects.

When I coached at the Stratford Festival, for example, an actor came to a tutorial extremely hoarse. The director had wanted a "strange" vocal quality, and the actor had attempted to create this quality by squeezing his tongue root and cutting off his breath. As a result, after 2 days of rehearsing with this tension, he was vocally tired. We experimented with using his nasal resonator and playing with the image of the sound emitting out of the bridge of his nose while paying special attention to his back rib support. Approaching the problem in this way allowed his tongue root, throat, and neck muscles to release and enabled him to gain full breath support, while still achieving the desired strange vocal quality. His voice regained its strength. Thus, the actor, vocal coach, and director were satisfied.

An actor recently came to me for a tutorial at Carnegie Mellon's School of Drama. He was learning the German accent and using the accent in a show as well. He was aware that he was vocally pushing. He was creating the guttural attack by tightening the muscles around his larynx. I suggested he think of getting the breath support fuller and thinking of the sound hitting the roof of his mouth (the hard palate), in the "mouth resonator." We also experimented with allowing his soft palate to loosen, to give a slight "guttural" quality. This allowed his larynx muscles to relax. This encouraged the sound to come "up and out" yet still create the desired guttural effect. Singers sometimes use the term *up and over the shelf*, referring to the image of thinking of the sound releasing up and over through the bone of the bottom of the skull, at the level of the nasal passages, above the hard palate.

Through proper technique, which includes appropriate breath support, placement, and use of resonators, the actor can find ways of producing sounds we would normally think of as unhealthy but do so in a reasonably healthy manner. There is always a little compromise, however, as it is extremely challenging to maintain such vocal choices for any length of time. The actor may end up pushing a little, but if he has done a sufficient warm-up before the performance and vocal cool-down afterwards, then he should be able to achieve the vocal choice without damage. If the actor connects strongly to the character's needs while incorporating physical ease, he should be able to integrate the technical demands effectively. In this circumstance, the actor needs to be particularly detailed in his text analysis. Sloppy text analysis, in any situation, often results in poor voice usage.

Directors and especially directing students should spend time analyzing voice usage by listening to television shows, movies, and plays and then describing what they hear. They should examine what "worked" vocally and what did not and why. Often audiences are aware that something the actor is doing is not affecting them deeply, but they do not understand why.

Some questions to bear in mind when viewing/listening:

- Is the actor's breath support efficient or does the actor use "top up" breathing, which is breathing primarily from the upper chest? Is there a sense that the breath releases easily with the sound and comes from the actor's whole body, or does the actor seem to tighten on the exhalation?

- Is the voice comfortable to listen to?

- Does the voice communicate nuances of character and emotion without strain?

- Does the actor "play" his voice, or does the voice usage merge fluidly with the character's intentions?

- Does the actor articulate self-consciously in a manner that brings our attention to his enunciation rather than to the ideas being communicated? Is the articulation integrated in such a way that the ideas are clarified and the actor uses the language to communicate the specifics of the intention?

- Does the actor's voice flow?
- Are the movement and the alignment integrated with the voice usage?
- Is the thought impulse propelling the sound?
- Does the actor's voice use seem spontaneous and effortless? (This is what we hope to achieve in any art form, as when the dancer makes the *tour jeté* seem easy—until we try it ourselves.)

In show business, many regard film acting as less vocally challenging than most stage acting. Many actors who work primarily in film do not devote a great deal of time or energy to voice training. Although film acting does not usually require the actor to vocally fill a large space, nonetheless the vocal demands in film, television, and other media can be taxing. Long shooting days and frequent takes of emotionally or physically challenging scenes can exhaust actors vocally and emotionally. Actors who are employed primarily in film and television should devote as much energy to voice training and maintaining vocal fitness as any stage actor. This will enable the film and television actor to be more versatile and flexible in choices of roles and able to switch effectively over to stage without having to "get back into shape vocally." Getting into top shape vocally can take several months and one doesn't want to be tackling challenging acting material while also getting into shape. Think of a dancer mastering a difficult choreography while attempting to build the strength, skill, and endurance necessary to support those moves.

Directors cognizant of the vocal challenges an actor faces in order to interpret a role possess the ability to support the actor through the rehearsal process. The director should develop sensitivity to situations in which the actor may be pushing vocally in order to gain a result too early in the rehearsal process. The director can increase his vocal awareness by listening to vocal qualities in actors playing in theater, film, television, radio, and voice-over. In the boxes are some helpful examples from film and television.

Examples of Healthy, Expressive, and Effective Voice Usage

Women

Angela Bassett in *Waiting to Exhale*

Kathy Bates in *Primary Colors*

Annette Bening in *Richard III* (with Ian McKellen)

Cate Blanchett in *An Ideal Husband*

Helena Bonham Carter in *Wings of the Dove*

Julie Christie in *Hamlet* (with Kenneth Branagh)

Martina Gedeck in *Mostly Martha*, *Das Leben der Anderen* (*The Lives of Others*)

Alison Jenney in *The West Wing*, *Primary Colors*

Helen Mirren in *The Queen*, *Gosford Park,* or anything

Kristin Scott Thomas in *Gosford Park*, *The English Patient*

Emma Thompson in *Primary Colors*

Sigourney Weaver in *Working Girl*

Dianne Wiest in *Bullets over Broadway*

Men

F. Murray Abraham in *Amadeus* (F. Murray Abraham's ability to make the language accessible and still maintain the elegant style of the period is particularly impressive here. His delivery in the role of Omar Suarez in *Scarface* is a nice contrast. Here the character is a rough, hyper underworld character with an entirely different vocal quality, still supported and clear, with a seamlessly integrated dialect.)

Alan Bates in *Hamlet* (with Mel Gibson)

Tom Cruise in *The Firm*

Billy Crystal in *Analyze This*

Daniel Day-Lewis in *The Boxer*, *The Name of the Father*

Robert De Niro in *Analyze This*

Leonardo di Caprio in *Catch Me If You Can*

Morgan Freeman in *The Shawshank Redemption*
Ed Harris in *The Firm*, *Glengarry Glen Ross*
Samuel L. Jackson in *Pulp Fiction*
Sebastian Koch in *Black Book*, *Das Leben der Anderen* (*The Lives of Others*)
Delroy Lindo in *Malcolm X*, *Cider House Rules*
Dylan McDermott in *The Practice*
Ian McKellen in *Richard III*, *Gods and Monsters*
Ulrich Mühe in *Das Leben der Anderen* (*The Lives of Others*)
Jeremy Northam in *The Winslow Boy*, *Gosford Park*
Laurence Olivier in *Henry V*
Al Pacino in *Glengarry Glen Ross*
Brad Pitt in *A River Runs Through It*
Liam Roache in *Priest*
Ulrich Tukur in *Das Leben der Anderen* (*The Lives of Others*)
Denzel Washington in *Malcolm X*

Controversial Voice Usage

Gary Oldman in *Dracula*
Chazz Palminteri in *Analyze This*
Billy Bob Thornton in *Sling Blade*

Examples of Unhealthy, Ineffective, and Inexpressive Voice Usage

It is interesting to note that many actors on this list are wonderful actors and in other examples use their voices effectively. Some are on both lists.

Men

Tom Cruise in *Interview with the Vampire* (When Mr. Cruise has the challenge of the dialect, he does not find the full-bodied ease of the character as he does in *The Firm*, so he strains his voice and his dialect is uneven.)

Leonardo DiCaprio in *Romeo and Juliet* (Here Mr. DiCaprio speaks with a great deal of vocal strain and lack of vocal clarity. A gifted actor, he would have benefited from the guidance of a voice/text coach in dealing with the challenges of the classical text.)

Brad Pitt in *Interview with the Vampire* (Mr. Pitt, again a gifted actor, spoke with strain, making the text muddled and unclear, particularly in emotional scenes.)

Giovanni Ribisi in *Boiler Room* (In many ways, a rich performance, but in the scene where he confronts his father, he works with enormous physical tension, particularly in the neck and shoulder area, and the voice quality becomes strangled as a result. This is in contrast with Ron Rifkin, who plays the father and manages to keep the stakes high in an intense emotional scene, but to stay grounded and free vocally.)

Women

Joey Lauren Adams in *Chasing Amy* (In this film, she works with so much vocal tension it is painful to watch the tight neck muscles, and difficult to listen to the strangled sound.)

Lara Flynn Boyle on *The Practice* (She is a strong actress, but pushes vocally, particularly in intense scenes.)

Glenn Close in *Hamlet* (with Mel Gibson) (Normally a wonderful actress, but in this Ms. Close is not comfortable with the language and sounds affected as a result. She tends to emotionalize in a way that makes her voice shrill sounding and disconnected.)

Meg Ryan in *Courage under Fire* (Ms. Ryan is usually a wonderfully relaxed actress, but in the scene in the helicopter, she is so intent on screaming rather than communicating her instructions that one cannot understand a word she is saying.

10 THE THOUGHT PROPELS THE SOUND

> In reality, such a character would want to make sure her precise instructions were being followed. Volume and emotion would be irrelevant. The actress got caught up in the externals and forgot what she was communicating and, therefore, so did we.)

Directors should familiarize themselves with voice vocabulary. *Off voice*, for example, refers to an overly breathy quality. It can communicate an affectation or a confidential, sexy quality. A good example is Anne Baxter as Eve Harrington in *All about Eve*. The off voice quality hints to us that the character is hiding something specific, or not fully revealing that she is. Some "soft sell" commercials (like for fleecy, soft tissue, etc.) use a breathy quality. This indicates the vocal folds are coming together without enough force (see Appendix). Marilyn Monroe was a master of the breathy sound to the point it really became her trademark, although probably a limiting one. Although it can be effective in certain situations, one wants to be judicious when employing off voice quality. It can tire the voice when overused, is difficult to sustain, and limits the ability of the actor to express the full depth and nuance of complex text.

A *squeezed* or *pushed* voice refers to a voice with an overbalance of voice production to the appropriate amount of breath, the other end of the spectrum from off voice. Some "hard sell" commercials utilize an overly pushed sound, such as Duracell battery commercials. A pushed or "pressed" sound indicates that the actor is producing sound with too much tension in the throat, pressing the vocal folds together with too much force on phonation, rather than using full breath support. When either quality is overused, listening to the actor can become grating. Generally, both extremes should be eschewed on stage because they tire the voice and do not allow the sound to carry fully. (See Appendix.)

Summary

Directors need to become listeners. They must develop the ability to discern the difference between expressive, clear, and healthy voice usage and unhealthy, garbled, and strangled voice usage. They need to analyze when an actor is misusing his or her voice and have strategies for guiding the actor to voice more effectively. Just as the opera director must understand music and qualities in singing, so the theater director must be attuned to the nuances and health of the actor's voice.

CHAPTER 2

Overview of Voice Methods: Whose Voice Is It Anyway?

*I*n the last century, various pedagogical philosophies and methods have influenced voice and speech training in acting programs in North America and overseas. Although a director may lack the time and resources to study every approach in depth, a director should at a minimum be familiar with the fundamentals of voice and speech training. The director who comprehends the nuances of voice, speech, and text as they relate to the actor's journey, with enough humility to recognize what she does not know, creates an environment in which actors can express themselves with vocal ease and confidence.

VOICE TRAINING

Training of the speaking voice usually refers to training in voice production. Vocal exercises, similar to those used in singing training, are employed to develop the full spectrum of the actor's range. These include exercises designed to:

- release physical tension;
- promote efficient breath support;

- release sound without constriction in the muscles of the laryngeal area;
- develop vocal stamina and dynamics, as well as flexibility of the articulators (soft palate, lips, tongue, jaw); and
- explore and strengthen awareness of resonating areas.

Sound vibrations resonate in the bones and tissue of the body primarily in the mask (sinus, cheekbones, bony area in the nose), skull, and chest/back areas. Tense muscles limit sound vibration; hence, the importance of relaxation in voice training.

Speech Training

Speech training involves the understanding of sound structures, and how to adapt these structures to various texts and dialects. In general, speech training centers on the shape/placement of articulators (lips, tongue, soft palate, and jaw) while making the sounds of language. The student learns to identify specific sounds relating to the appropriate symbol in the International Phonetic Alphabet (or some variation thereof) much as a musician learns to identify specific musical notes to particular symbols in sheet music. In prescriptive approaches, the student learns these sounds and symbols while, at the same time, mastering a "standard" dialect of North American speech or in the UK, standard British, also termed Received Pronunciation. Traditional speech training generally focuses on the external and more technical aspects of speaking, for example, how to shape a particular sound, what inflection to use, which words to emphasize. This kind of speech training places more emphasis on the "auditory" aspects of learning: "How does that sound?" "Can you hear the difference?"

Speaking voice training, on the other hand, generally focuses on voice production and the kinesthetic relationship to sound and language: "Where do you sense this in your body? What do the sound vibrations feel like?" Ideally, training should incorporate and integrate both aspects of learning. The great pioneer in voice/speech training approaches, Cicely Berry (Officer of the British Empire and Director of Voice at the Royal Shakespeare Company in England), creatively combines both these aspects. She has devised explorations that sensitize the actor to the relationship of meaning, sound, and vocal ease. The connection among the kinesthetic experiences of sound, the inherent rhythm of language, and how these aspects shape meaning at a deeper visceral level form an essential component of actor training. Ideally, all voice and speech work should link to acting text from the onset of training.

The physical aspects of voice training follow a progression much like the training of an athlete. However, voice training differs from the training of the athlete in a significant respect: the actor needs to coordinate the physical aspects of the training with the impulse of thought within the actor. The actor must engage her imagination in order to pursue the intention of the character as written. The actor must then integrate these to impact another actor/character on stage.

This delicate interplay of imagination and technical demands challenges teacher and student alike. The overall mechanism of the speaking voice involves all facets of the individual: intellectual, psychological, physiological, spiritual, as well as anatomical. The study becomes intensely personal in some respects, sometimes even more so than other aspects of actor training. The physical voice in its ease, dynamic, and flexibility reflects the inner workings of the individual, what Cicely Berry refers to as "that secret voice" (Berry, 2000). Each actor is unique and needs a different balance of emphasis in her training and coaching. Training may, therefore, incorporate personal writing and therapeutic techniques as tools to open up the full range of the actor's vocal experience both in the practical and in the metaphorical sense. The metaphorical sense refers to the actor tapping into her need to free her own unique vocal expression. The teacher provides a map but the student takes the internal journey. Most teachers teach what worked best for them in their own training, which explains why a number of approaches exist. It behooves the teacher to familiarize himself with a variety of pedagogical methods to tailor coaching to best suit individual actor needs. That said, the student needs to master certain fundamentals, involving the daily discipline of practicing a proper vocal warm-up to maintain vocal stamina, breath support, resonance, clear articulation, and so on, much along the lines of regular scales for the pianist or a ballet *barre* for the ballet dancer. When the teacher creates a non-judgmental atmosphere, with the appropriate rigor, the possibilities for vocal growth increase.

KRISTIN LINKLATER'S PSYCHOPHYSICAL APPROACH

There exist a number of speaking voice training methods in North America. One of the most established is the approach developed first by Iris Warren at Central School of Speech and Drama in London, England, and brought to the United States by Kristin Linklater in 1963 when she established a studio in New York City. She taught at New York University and coached for the Working Theatre and later the Open Theatre with Joe Chaikin and Sam Shepard. As regional theaters developed across North America, it became apparent that many actors did not possess adequate vocal training needed to fill larger theater spaces and to handle the diverse vocal demands asked of an actor in a repertory season. In 1965, in order to help address this need, Linklater began training teachers in her method. Her first group of teacher trainees included a number of now well-established voice teachers: David Smukler (Head of Voice, York University), Fran Bennett (former Head of Acting, California Institute of the Arts), and Dudley Knight (former Vice Chair, Drama, University of California, Irvine). Since that period, Linklater has continued to train teachers on a regular basis both in the United States and internationally, including regular teacher training programs in Germany.

In 1990, Linklater developed a Linklater Designation to distinguish people who may be familiar with her method from those whose training she has personally supervised. In the training, Linklater emphasizes the importance of modeling the work effectively as one teaches. The Linklater teacher should exemplify a strong psychophysical awareness as she teaches and the sense of being fully authentic and "present." Sometimes voice/speech trainers develop a "teacher" voice, using the voice to mask expression, creating an affectation rather than engaging the voice to reveal more deeply the authentic self. In a learning situation, teaching, and/or professional coaching, it is important that the voice coach model healthy, effective, and expressive voice usage. A coach may teach an actor the most fantastic exercises, but if the coach cannot embody the principles of the psychophysical work, the work will have little impact.

Many training programs make use of Linklater's book *Freeing the Natural Voice* published by Drama Publishers in 1976 with an excellent revision in 2006. Kristin Linklater has taught and coached internationally and, in 1978, she and Tina Packer founded Shakespeare

& Company in Lenox, Massachusetts. Shakespeare & Company was one of the first companies in the United States to employ interracial casting, which at the time was considered quite radical. This, fortunately, is no longer the case. Linklater left Shakespeare & Company in the late 1980s to teach full-time at Emerson College in Boston. Linklater is now professor at Columbia University's theater division Master's of Fine Arts Program, where she heads the acting program.

Linklater has conducted workshops with Carol Gilligan, author of *In a Different Voice* (1982), which deals with the silencing of young women in our society. Gilligan's book examines how young women are discouraged from expressing themselves, particularly as they enter adolescence. It also investigates the strength of young women's interpersonal and collaborative skills, pointing out that these skills are not highly valued in our culture. As a manifestation of this silencing, young women tend to become weak vocally. Linklater and Gilligan have developed a number of explorations, including personal writing, to help young women connect more fully to their creative voices and vocal power, as these relate to their emotional lives. From this work, Linklater went on to develop The Company of Women, a group of actresses devoted to producing all-female versions of Shakespeare productions. They also give workshops helping women "find their voices" in the fullest sense. The Company of Women works out of Boston, New York, and Los Angeles.

The Linklater-trained actor examines his or her own psyche in relation to the voice and text work. The philosophical basis of the technique challenges the student to address her own emotional blocks, reflecting a more radical political point of view. The intimate association of freeing the voice and how the voice work impacts the emotional life of the actor makes up a significant component of the Linklater training. As Linklater writes in *Freeing the Natural Voice*, "The natural voice is transparent—revealing, not describing, inner impulses of emotion and thought, directly and spontaneously. The *person* is heard, not the person's *voice*" [my italics] (Linklater, revised 2006, p. 8).

The Linklater exercises follow a systematic progression, each sequence organically building to warm up the whole vocal apparatus while working gently to deepen breath support as one stimulates the imagination and emotional center. The system thoroughly addresses tension in the lips, jaw, soft palate, tongue, and tongue root, releasing laryngeal tension. Tensions in these areas stifle a free, open, forward sound. Some methods attempt to address breath support, while not successfully releasing the jaw, tongue, soft palate, and tongue root tension. This results in a "forced" support and a pushed, tense sound caused by tightness in the muscles around the larynx, soft palate, jaw, and tongue. Linklater's method is extremely effective in releasing tension in these areas. Another strength of the approach is the text and voice exercises, with a strong sound and movement basis, detailed in Linklater's *Freeing Shakespeare's Voice* (1992).

The Linklater work is solidly grounded in the relationship of the voice, the body, and the person—or the psychophysical aspects of the work. As a result, the Linklater-trained actor tends to connect well in her body, with a good intuitive relationship to text. Some Linklater teachers overemphasize the emotional relationship to text, which can lead to a phenomenon that Linklater herself refers to as *excitation*, that is, when the emotional response to the text overwhelms the clarity. The actor can become seduced by her "feelings," which can obscure meaning and short-change the full exploration of the specific thoughts and intentions. This emphasis on feelings often takes the actor away from her full support, causing tightening in the throat. As a director or voice/text coach, one needs to remind the actor to pay attention to the clarity of thoughts as well as the intentions of the character, so these lead the speaking of text, rather than allowing the emotions to dominate the speaking. The actor needs to focus on the ladder of the thoughts (that is, the way in which the argument builds, as this allows the voice to respond to and reflect the build of ideas) rather than pushing for a particular end result of emotion. When the thoughts and intentions lead, the emotional response to the language actually occurs simultaneously with the thought and does not impede clarity. The actor, however, does not need to concern herself with the emotion, only with the intention and the thoughts. The actor needs to maintain enough psychophysical ease to release the thoughts and to remain true to the intent of the character when a genuine emotional response is triggered by the strength of the language and the dramatic situation of the character. This is where the importance of voice, speech, and Alexander work comes to the fore, as it gives the actor the ability to remain open and release into the ideas and demands of the text, rather than responding to the text by squeezing and pulling down physically and vocally, which prevents the full expression of the text.

Linklater's work is taught at Columbia University, New York University, Carnegie Mellon, Yale, University of California in Los Angeles, Cal Arts, York University, and many other training programs. The training emphasizes a flexible, expressive body, the release of sound with ease, with a relaxed method of support while developing a deeply kinesthetic relationship to language. The Linklater-trained actor should also possess the ability to successfully tackle classical texts, new plays, as well as experimental and physically challenging theater.

CATHERINE FITZMAURICE: DESTRUCTURING AND RESTRUCTURING

Another method of voice training now established in the United States is the Fitzmaurice approach, developed by Catherine Fitzmaurice, also a graduate of the Central School of Speech and Drama, where she trained with Barbara Bunch and Cicely Berry. When she came to the United States, she observed that American actors had a strong emotional connection to text but often were less specific in terms of text analysis and support than their British counterparts. The British actors, on the other hand, grasped text analysis and the ability to fill a large space but frequently without a deeper emotional connection to the language. Fitzmaurice has coached and trained some of our most accomplished actors, having held consulting and teaching appointments at University of Delaware, Central School of Speech and Drama, Juilliard School, Yale University, Harvard/Moscow Art Theatre, the Guthrie Theater, Lincoln Center, and a number of other training programs, as well as running a studio for a number of years in Los Angeles and now in New York City. Over a number of years, she explored bioenergetics, yoga, and other body modalities and integrated these with the voice work. She terms these aspects of her approach *destructuring* work. She combines these with the work of Clifford Turner, with whom she studied in England. Fitzmaurice refers to Turner's *rib reserve* technique as the *restructuring* aspect of the work.

As with Linklater's approach, the Fitzmaurice voice work involves the actor exploring emotional release as it relates to the body through the restructuring process, using the bioenergetics and yoga positions. Each position creates a tension/release situation in the body, often resulting in a *tremor*—the same principle as when we overwork a muscle and it quakes and the shaking we experience when we sob deeply, shiver, orgasm, and so on. This primitive release allows the breath to deepen and the voice to open more fully. Each position is designed to address specific areas in the body that are likely to block the breath flowing freely. This aspect of the method is dramatic and exciting, enabling the actor to touch emotional reservoirs. The body is then ready for the restructuring process. This involves expanding the intercostals muscles, with particular emphasis on the initial expanse of the back ribs as the breath comes in, maintaining that position until the breath/sound releases. A criticism of the old rib reserve was that the actor became rigid in her delivery. Combined with the destructuring process, however, the rib reserve can provide excellent breath support, as over time one learns to swing the ribs with ease. One is able to adapt the rib reserve to allow for more flexibility as well as a visceral and expressive connection to text. In my own experience, I integrate this work with the Alexander Technique and find the students develop a full-bodied support, enabling them to tackle any performance challenge, while maintaining psychophysical freedom, without stiffness.

There are differences between the philosophies of Fitzmaurice's and Linklater's work (most notably in the approach to breath support) though, in my experience, they are quite compatible. Fitzmaurice breath support is more rigorous and athletic and particularly good for dealing with heightened moments in acting. The Linklater work is particularly valuable at the onset of training, to ground the breath and the actor and to raise the actor's consciousness about the experience of psychophysical vocal work in general. The Fitzmaurice work can threaten the more inhibited individual and therefore is often more successfully incorporated once the student has mastered the basics of kinesthetic voice work and the actor has become reasonably secure in her foundation As with the Linklater approach, because the work interplays so much with the actor's psyche, the actor can make the faulty assumption that if she is "feeling," no other work is required. The actor must constantly remember to bring the work back to the text. At Carnegie Mellon, this method is introduced at the 3rd year level of the BFA acting training, once the student has begun to master the basics of the Linklater voice work. It is often difficult for students to understand that voice work takes several years and can be repetitive in its nature. The Fitzmaurice work provides a nice challenge and change of pace well suited to the more advanced stages of the actor's undergraduate training though certainly quite appropriate for the onset of a graduate vocal training program.

When I first completed my Fitzmaurice training, I was coaching a show at Pittsburgh Public Theater. I was particularly proud of my warm-up designed especially for the company, combining a synthesis of the work of Linklater, Fitzmaurice, and Cicely Berry. One cast member had trained with Catherine Fitzmaurice and during the warm-up became extremely vocal in her sounds, which sounded like she was having a rather dramatic orgasm. The next day, I was about to start the warm-up, always a slightly nervous moment for a coach in a professional situation. The director came to me and whispered in my ear, "Janet, can you please cut the 'shaky' stuff? I would be afraid to be in a dark room with that one [referring to the actress]!" An actress I worked with many years ago at the Stratford Festival gave me some good advice: Never argue with the person signing your paycheck. So I made the appropriate adjustments while still incorporating the principles of the work.

As with all systems, however, the director must constantly remind the actor to go for her intention. The more the director understands the rigors of text work, of course, the more the director will help the actor find specifics in the text.

Fitzmaurice's work, although still considered controversial by some, is now well established and taught at many of the top training institutions across the United States including Carnegie Mellon, the University of California at Irvine, the University of Delaware, Yale, Juilliard, and the American Repertory Theatre/Moscow Art Theatre program at Harvard. It is particularly valuable for actors who have been trained in the more rigid approaches to speech as it helps them loosen up and develop a more organic connection to language.

ARTHUR LESSAC'S VOICE TRAINING

Arthur Lessac began his well-known Lessac Kinesensic Training for the voice and body in 1937. One aspect of his method approaches sounds in a kinesthetic manner, exploring them as if each were a musical instrument in an orchestra. He has taught internationally and for many years at the State University of New York (SUNY) and his work is the focus of the Lessac Training and Research Institute, which offers regular workshops for actors, lay people, and teachers. He has influenced and trained many voice teachers, including Bonnie Raphael and master Lessac teacher Deborah Kinghorn, who is collaborating with Lessac on his third book. For more information, see Resources for a listing of his publications and website.

ROBERT PARKS' JOURNEY

Robert Parks taught at Carnegie Mellon for 25 years. His initial training began with Edith Skinner. He worked as a professional actor, and then proceeded to study speech pathology, singing, Feldenkrais, tai chi, and the Alexander Technique to develop his method called *The Journey*. In this method, the actor goes through a series of tai chi style movements. A specific image and sound are assigned to each movement, such as "smelling flower," "flying eagle," and "chopping wood." The series progresses systematically, beginning gently and becoming more vigorous as it evolves. The imagery use sparks the actor's imagination as the vocal warm-up develops. The technique provides the actor with a solid vocal preparation, which adapts well to different acting demands. Robert Parks, who now lives in Maine, is writing a book about his method.

ROY HART'S EXTENDED VOICE

Roy Hart (a British actor) and Alfred Volsen (a German musician) developed the Roy Hart extended voice approach. Volsen had survived the trenches of World War I in Germany and was amazed at the sounds that came out of his fellow soldiers as they were dying. After the war, Volsen explored whether one could develop these extreme sounds and extended pitches through joy and artistic expression. Volsen and Roy Hart started a company in England, which later relocated to the south of France. The company performed experimental works that allowed the actors to explore extreme vocal expression.

After Hart and his wife died suddenly in a plane crash in 1975, the company floundered for a time but now has a center in France, which offers certification in this work. Roy Hart's son Jonathan Hart and his colleague Richard Armstrong (one of the founding members of the Roy Hart Company) teach in New York City and give workshops internationally. (For more information, see Resources.)

The Roy Hart methods emphasize a great deal of freedom, vocal flexibility, and fearlessness. Proponents of this method claim the ability to reach a range of up to five octaves and believe that this is within the potential of every human voice. When the Roy Hart group first started, there were rumors that the actors had had vocal implants put into their larynxes to enable them to achieve this kind of range![1]

There is a great deal of exploration of resonance in different parts of the body, through character work. For example, when using the chest/mouth area the actor plays the role of a diva opera singer and for the nasal and upper mask area, she takes on the role of an evil elf. The extended voice work enriches an actor's (and singer's) vocal repertoire. The approach tends toward bold, emotional strokes and must be tackled rather carefully, so as not to overextend the voice so much that the actor risks vocal strain or injury. From the director's perspective, the actor integrating this method with text may need reminders to stay specific in terms of the ladder of thought and go "moment to moment," rather than approaching text in generalized "chunks."

THE VOICE AND EMOTION

Many of the psychophysical approaches incorporate therapeutic approaches and personal writing work. If a person is terribly blocked emotionally, then psychophysical voice work may be quite threatening. The actor needs a considerable amount of self-awareness and courage to embark on this aspect of the vocal journey. As the actor delves more deeply into the voice work, generally she will find certain emotional connections to the work, some of which may be painful or frightening. Sometimes, during a voice class or

---

[1]Conversations with Richard Armstrong at the Banff Center for the Arts, Banff, Canada, 1996.

even after a session, people may feel quite vulnerable, cry, laugh, feel irritable, frightened, and a whole gamut of other emotional responses. Sometimes individuals experience nausea and/or dizziness. This can result from the person taking in more oxygen than usual, or it can simply be a psychophysical response to the vulnerability of the work itself. Given the nature of the work, some voice teachers set themselves up as therapist or guru, which is not helpful to actors. One of the aspects of Cicely Berry's work I admire is that she allows the actor space to respond to the work, which may occasionally result in an emotional response, but she doesn't impose this on the actor. She lets the actor make the discovery absolutely on her own, thereby letting the actor own the response. If an actor becomes emotional, the best thing is to get onto text immediately. I remember Kristin Linklater telling a group of actors at a Shakespeare & Company workshop, "Whatever you are feeling, put it into the Shakespeare text—it can hold all of it." As a voice/speech teacher, one may occasionally need to suggest someone see a counselor if the work is stirring up a lot of issues that make it difficult for the actor to pursue the work effectively. If the actor experiences emotion that appears to be overwhelming the actor, a director (or acting/voice coach) might want to ask him if he is comfortable continuing or whether he needs a break. If the scene is particularly emotional, it might be a good idea to allow a little debriefing time before going on to the next scene.

When I studied, I always cried when we worked on the sinus resonator. I do not know exactly why, but I am surmising it was something to do with a dropped soft palate (a common occurrence when one has grown up in Montreal, where one hears French so much as French has many nasal sounds in which the soft palate is dropped), which caused my voice to not resonate much in my face. I believe this became a rather protective mask as an adolescent, and when I began opening up vocally in that area, some of the feelings that the physical block protected in the first place brought the tears to the surface. Interestingly enough, I have taught this resonator now for many years and I do not get emotional when I teach it. When I study and am back in the role of a student, however, I, once again, become emotionally vulnerable when working in this resonating area. Our psychophysical makeup is extremely complex!

A number of years ago, I decided to separate the men and women in voice class in their third year at Carnegie Mellon's School of Drama when I introduced the Fitzmaurice voice work. This work challenges the students both technically and emotionally. The gender-specific groups provided an easier atmosphere for these young adults, and I was quite stunned at how much each group improved, both genders, as compared to previous years. During that year, I arranged a meeting with women faculty and students to discuss issues dealing with nudity and sexuality on stage, which had been causing anxiety for various students in rehearsal. Some of the women were shy to say when they felt uncomfortable in a rehearsal situation. One of the students, the talented and highly intelligent Paloma Guzman, spoke up and said, "Well a lot of the confidence to express when one is uncomfortable has to do with one's sense of having the right to speak. We have been studying voice this year with the men and women in separate groups. We women are really finding out about our right to speak, to use our voices and how to express our sense of entitlement through the voice work." I couldn't have paid her to express my goals more clearly! I am not saying men and women should always be trained separately, of course, but for a portion of the training, this can prove extremely helpful. This is another example of how the voice work is intrinsically connected with the whole person.

The ideal in training is to create an atmosphere where, if someone needs to release an emotion, she can do so with relative safety. On the other hand, it is not appropriate for teachers to push actors into an emotional release or manipulate actors into this as voice or acting teachers sometimes do. I am aware of an acting teacher who asked everyone in a class to call an African American the *N* word, because she was attempting to get him angry in a scene. In another workshop, a man had a glass eye, and the teacher asked everyone to point at it and to heckle the actor, in order to get the actor angry. At the end of the workshop, the poor man said to me, "I really don't know what has happened to me." This kind of treatment is absolutely inappropriate and potentially damaging psychologically.

I participated in a workshop once in which the voice teacher spoke about the connection of sexual abuse and the voice, explaining that sometimes when one finds a deeper connection to the breath, there can be a strong emotional response if one has experienced sexual abuse. A woman in the class let out a blood-curdling scream at the top of her lungs. The teacher just continued speaking as if nothing had happened as the woman ran out of the room howling. On the other end of the spectrum, I have worked with teachers who would have chased after her yelling, "Who are you angry at?" Somewhere, there is a balance of acknowledging that the voice relates to emotion, and supporting an actor through it without emotionally violating the actor.

THE VOICE AND WRITING

Writing helps to channel emotional feelings that voice work may trigger. During my training with Kristin Linklater, we wrote poems to our voices, as if the voice were a person or an entity one could talk to, and then worked on these pieces from a dramatic point of view. We also created "river stories," a variety of writing exercises including a monologue, a song, a scene, and a poem performed in groups. These were inspiring ways to explore the voice. I assign the voice poem exercise with a slight adaptation of writing a letter to one's voice. One can have actors draw a picture of the voice. In the Resonex chapter, the reader will find outlined various ways to incorporate writing with the exploration of resonators.

Cicely Berry has led numerous workshops on voice and writing, including workshops in prisons. She actually mentored one of the prisoners to write a play, which was produced at the RSC.

For the last nine years, the late Professor Milan Stitt, author of *The Runner Stumbles* (1976) and Head of Playwriting in the School of Drama at Carnegie Mellon University, and I team taught a project entitled "Monomania." I began by guiding the students through a number of free-flow writing exercises based on the exercises in Natalie Goldberg's *Writing Down the Bones: Freeing the Writer Within* (1986) and *Wild Mind: Living the Writer's Life* (1990) and a writing workshop I took with Lisa Kron, a member of the theater company Five Lesbian Brothers. Then Stitt would teach the students about monologue structure and, once the students had written their monologues, would give them feedback on their writing. I would spend a few weeks coaching them on integrating the voice and acting work with the monologue and occasionally send them back to Stitt for help with the writing. Then the monologues were performed for the school. The students often took huge leaps in the voice work in terms of finding more vocal range, resonance, vocal freedom, and flexibility. Once these qualities were tapped, the student could then begin to integrate them into their explorations with other text, particularly classical such as Greek, Shakespeare, Shaw, and the like. The interesting thing about these original monologues was that whatever the vocal challenge of the particular student, the student invariably wrote a monologue that forced him to tackle that vocal issue or the monologue would not succeed. For example, if the student tended to rush and had poor articulation, the monologue she wrote required precise clarity to play effectively. Or if the actor was challenged in terms of breath support, she would write something that was so powerful in terms of the character's need that the actor absolutely had to support the voice for the piece to work. I never mentioned this paradox to them, so it is not as if the students were deliberately looking for this result by any means. It is as if the inner creative soul actually knew exactly where it needed to go.

The project has allowed many students who did not realize they had a writing talent to discover that indeed they do. Several have used their monologue for the showcase in New York and Los Angeles, such as Paul Linquist and Katie Rogal, and a few—such as Gaius Charles, Ashley Sherman, Corey Moosa, and Kylee Rousselot—have been inspired to develop one-person shows. Brian Shoaf was in the first junior class to do this project and since he has written novels, screenplays, and plays and completed his MFA in playwriting at University of California, Los Angeles.

GOALS IN VOICE TRAINING

In training, the goal is to provide a strong technical basis, a fully engaged psychophysical connection to breath, sound, thought, and the word, as well as a sense of ownership in the voice work. Toward this end, I use a number of projects at Carnegie Mellon and UCLA. One is entitled Monomania, described above, and another is the Original Resonex described in Chapter 6.

Another project, which has proven enormously successful in training students at Carnegie Mellon, is an independent voice project I've nicknamed the INDIE project. Each student is assigned to give a short background on an aspect of voice based on a chapter in *The*

Vocal Vision (Hampton & Acker, 2000; see References) and develop and lead a practical experiential workshop for the class. Topics have included Emotion and Voice, Self-Esteem and Voice, Voice and Text Explorations, Sense Exploration and Voice/Text, Voice and Depression, Voice and Eating Disorders, Care of the Voice (dealing with reflux, nodes, etc.), and many others topics. Here I include some examples: Vicki Ward led a workshop experimenting with the impact of gospel singing on text and the ideas from *A Practical Handbook for the Actor* (Vintage, 1986); Kellie Goode explored how painting impacts text delivery; Emma Galvin experimented with how listening to different kinds music influenced the delivery; Nick Lehane experimented with the difference between focusing on communicating or playing acting objectives; other projects included mindful eating and its impact on voice (Steffie Garrard, Zach Berger, and Ethan Saks); riffing and its impact on spoken text (Zak Resnick, Brittany Campbell, and Mathenee Treco); history and practice of Roy Hart Voice Work (Shelby Lewis); the application of Fitzmaurice work on singing; utilizing concepts from Joan Melton's *One Voice* (2000, listed in the back under Resources); text explorations inspired by Cicely Berry's *Text in Action* (2000); and numerous others.

A few great things happen with this project. The students gain a broader understanding of the limitless extent of the voice world, enabling them to think about voice beyond the classroom. They also discover how much they have learned and mastered during the course of their training. When each student gives her presentation, invariably she is on voice and taking her vocal and physical space, gaining a wonderful sense of ownership about the work.

SUMMARY

The psychophysical voice work is an essential building block in an actor's development of an organic approach that includes a deep connection of the voice with the whole person and with the actor's creativity. It allows the actor to develop a visceral connection to sound, language, and intention, thereby bringing a full-blooded actor to performance.

If one were to develop a scale of expressiveness for methods of voice training, *organic* describes the work of Robert Parks' The Journey; *connected*, Linklater's work; *expansive*, Fitzmaurice's work; *vigorous* for the Lessac work; and perhaps *wanton* for the Roy Hart work. All these methods aim to release the inner impulse of speaking text in a way that engages the full mind, body, and imagination.

Some of the methods incorporate therapeutic approaches, but it is important to emphasize that release of emotion, although satisfying for an actor, and arguably an important aspect of the actor's training, does not satisfy an audience. What the actor *feels* is irrelevant. It is what the actor *does* in pursuit of her action that allows the audience to fully engage.

Directors and voice coaches should tread with caution when adapting therapeutic methods to voice and acting training and should avoid setting themselves up as gurus and/or therapists. Training programs for directing should include a minimum of a year of voice training in at least some of these approaches in order to properly prepare the director for her career. Psychophysical methods, sanely and respectfully approached, however, are most helpful to the actor's training because they encourage the deep connection of the actor to her body, cognition, and imagination.

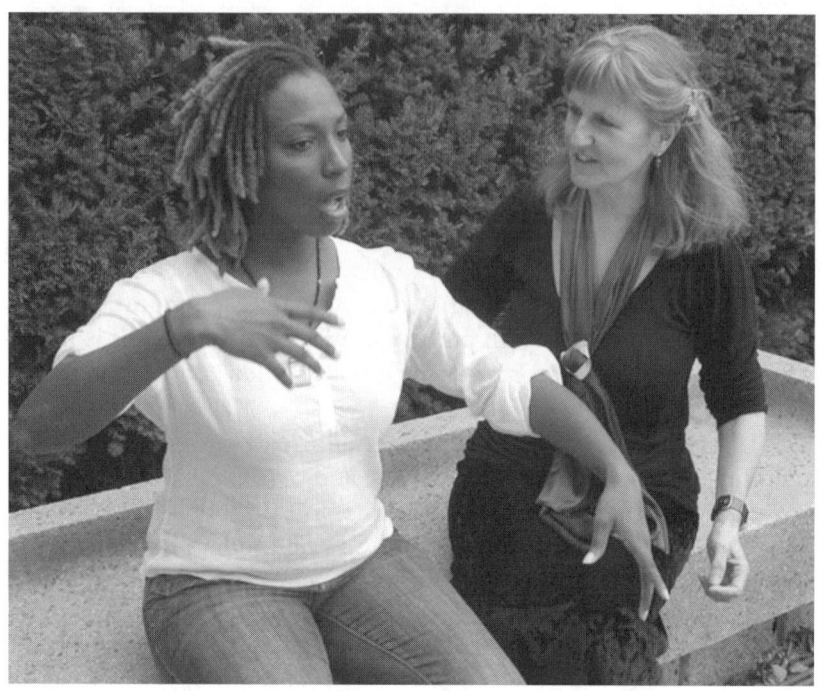
Left to right, Roberta Burke (BFA, Acting, School of Drama, Carnegie Mellon, 2009) and Janet Madelle Feindel (author). Photo by Karen Waggoner.

CHAPTER 3

Overview of Speech Methods: Whose Standard Is It Anyway?

THE SPEECH WORK

My early voice training focused primarily on Linklater voice work and the work of Robert Palmer at the Royal Academy of Dramatic Art. It was not until I began to teach voice that I investigated speech and phonetics training, initially while doing a teacher training with David Smukler. While on faculty at Kent State University's School of Theatre, I studied phonetics (from quite a different perspective) through the speech pathology department at Kent State with Dr. Richard Klick to facilitate a dialects course I was assigned to teach. At Carnegie Mellon, I encountered the Skinner method to "good American stage speech" in much more depth, which has been taught there for many years. I also studied the method in detail. Good American stage speech tends toward a "mid-Atlantic" sound in which certain British sounds are mixed with an American dialect. In order to gain an understanding of the dialect, the reader might listen to some old Lauren Bacall, Bette Davis, and Katherine Hepburn movies and observe the characteristics. Over the last decade, most theaters adopt what we normally term a more *general American* sound. In other words, for the most part it is no longer fashionable for American or Canadian actors to sound British or mid-Atlantic.

However, some training programs still teach the mid-Atlantic approach. Some actors, coaches, and directors still believe one cannot speak Shakespeare without employing a mid-Atlantic sound. This is unfortunate because this approach, particularly when started too early in the actor's training, can create a number of vocal issues. Actors tend to tighten vocally in order to achieve the required sounds and/or get *off voice*. Off voice refers to when an actor becomes breathy or emits a "shallow" sound that is not fully supporting the voice but speaking with limited physical connection. The sound becomes a way of masking the authentic self rather than allowing the voice to reveal a deeper connection to the soul of the character.

The accomplished and talented American actor, F. Murray Abraham, aptly elaborates: "Like Joseph Papp, I was a vigorous crusader for Shakespeare with an American accent . . . I don't think any actor can give an honest performance of anything while impersonating someone else. If Shakespeare is as universal as everyone says, then let his words be spoken the way I speak . . . [American actors] become weird around Shakespeare, their bodies stiffen, their voices change, and they start to sing their lines . . . " (Abraham, 2005, p. 6).

Once these bad habits become established, it becomes difficult to overcome them.

Initially, speech training focused on "elocution," but nowadays one wants to incorporate as much of a kinesthetic approach to speech training as one can. One wants also to involve the whole psychophysical system of the actor, so that the speech work always reflects the clarity of thought and the intention. Newer systems to speech training offer much more inclusive approaches in terms of diversity, so that the standard American speech model is not used as a tool to imply the way the student speaks habitually is somehow inherently bad. The standard American dialect is simply an option an actor should be familiar with, as it gives an actor more choices. The teacher can approach the dialect creatively in a variety of ways, for example by helping students identify each other's speech sounds without judging what makes a "good" or "bad" sound allows the students to explore the way sounds are formed, exploring their kinesthetic sense. This helps create an atmosphere where all backgrounds are valued. Using diverse texts for speech work reinforces a more inclusive approach as well. One can, for example, use the speeches of Martin Luther King, Jr., Malcolm X, Germaine Greer, or Sojourner Truth instead of the traditional and often-outdated speech ditties such as "Peter Piper picked a peck of pickled peppers," etc. Speech training should not be taught in a mechanical way but rather in a manner that engages the actor's imagination. Speech is often taught through mechanical articulation drills but this is counterproductive to actor training. Repeating mindless drills removes the imagination and thought component and thus trains the psychophysical mechanism to detach from the thought and imagination, rather than integrate these more fully into the process. And this is exactly what we do *not* want to reinforce in actors. What needs developing is the intricate psychophysical interplay of the thought, imagination, and communication with the breath impulse, movement of the intercostal muscles and diaphragm, full sense of the body, and the shaping of sound (thoughts) with the articulatory muscles. In other words, speech training needs to reinforce the actor's ability to form images and ideas in the mind and connect these thoughts and images in a kinesthetic manner. This is a challenging task at the best of times, so one needs to buttress this as much as possible.

Voice and speech teachers (as well as acting teachers and directors) need to employ positive teaching methods if they wish to create an inclusive atmosphere and help actors fully utilize their full sound and range. If you speak with a Texas drawl, this should be viewed as an asset, not a problem to "correct." Urban myth states that Edith Skinner told the young Holly Hunter that Ms. Hunter would *never* work if she did not rid herself of her Texas dialect. A talented young actress I coached in New York told me about her first encounter with speech class when she arrived to study at a prestigious New York City acting program. After the speech teacher heard her speak with her native Texas dialect, he rolled his eyes and mimed rolling up his sleeves and heaved a sigh followed by "Have we got our work cut out for us." The actress told me she had felt demeaned and "labeled" after she had barely opened her mouth. How much tension does that create in a young actor before she has even begun the work?

A number of years ago I taught a talented actor, an African American young man, who did an independent project for the class in which he taught the class Ebonics with the premise that this should be the standard American dialect. Whether one agrees or not with his proposition, it provoked a lively discussion. Shouldn't these discussions be part of actor training? It seems some training programs are afraid to let actors question and actually think about how voice and speech reflect the political and sociological aspects of the times and how this impacts pedagogy. Don't we want to encourage actors to lead and challenge rather than train them to be complacent and obedient? It is clear that there is quite a range in what is considered "standard American." Language breathes and evolves, so the standard in the 1930s and 1940s is not the standard today. The standard generally represents the ruling class, but given that the last two presidents spoke with variations of a southern dialect and these days it seems fashionable for politicians to drop their "g" sounds at the ends of words ending in "ing," perhaps that might be closer to what we presume as a "standard"!

A gifted young actor I recently coached in New York told me that in the last show he had acted in, the coach criticized him after the first reading, telling him he should pitch his voice differently. A first reading is generally far too early to be giving notes, particularly such an external note that has little to do with the context of the play or, more specifically, the intention of the character. Good acting requires flexibility, imagination, and humor. Speech teaching and coaching need to incorporate that same flexibility and sense of inquiry and humor in order to truly educate the actor and support him in his process.

It's important that directors realize that many actors come with "voice and speech" baggage if actors have experienced shame-based training. For example, I have had actors looking terrified and shuddering as they tell me, "I am nasal." Nasality is not a character defect. It simply reflects a tight soft palate and plenty of exercises are available to address that. Although of course actors want the option of not being nasal, many good actors are nasal and have had quite successful careers: Jack Nicholson and Maggie Smith, to name but two.

Every actor's dialect is valid and a great starting point. Of course, over time an actor needs to develop options and flexibility. In a conversation during rehearsals of *The Merchant of Venice* with F. Murray Abraham, an actor renowned for his mellifluous voice and clear diction, he told me his native dialect, a combination of Texas and Hispanic, was the one he used for the character he played in *Scarface*. What a great asset his natural affinity for that dialect was for a brilliant and completely believable interpretation of the role! Again, the point is to encourage actors to have options rather than creating a system of correct and incorrect ways of speaking.

Some actors seem to be speech-proof and director-proof, but many talented actors, capable of strong engaging performances, are not. I worked with a wonderful actress who became completely undermined at a major Shakespeare festival because of constant negative feedback about her voice from the artistic director and the voice and speech coach. This rarely helps the actor to improve but often serves only to make him self-conscious—and self-consciousness is the enemy of all good acting. Several actors I have coached related similar traumatic experiences in their training that left them undermined, even years later. Sadly this kind of early negative experience can render the actor defensive and incapable or unwilling to address legitimate voice and speech issues that limit their careers.

PRESCRIPTIVE APPROACHES

The Traditional Skinner Approach: History and Necessary Evolution

Edith Warman Skinner was one of the strongest influences on American speech training. She trained a generation of actors and many speak of her in reverential terms. Edith Skinner studied with Margaret Prendergast McLean, who in turn had trained with William Tilly, an Australian phonetician. Tilly came to New York City in 1918, where he took a teaching position at Columbia University. His students consisted of pupils learning English as a second language as well as teachers in the public school system who desired to maintain "acceptable" standards of English pronunciation. Tilly employed the phonetic alphabet that at the time was evolving as a tool used in anthropology and linguistics to notate sounds. He initially used the *broad phonetics* adopted by the International Phonetics Association, founded in 1880 by the Frenchman Paul Passy. Tilly went further by developing *narrow* phonetic transcription, which consisted of more detailed transcription, using various diacritic symbols. His main interest was teaching English as a spoken language, rather than as a written language, using the International Phonetic Alphabet as a tool.

Although Tilly himself did not possess a huge interest in the theater, a number of his students went on to influence American theater voice and speech training. One was Windsor P. Daggett. He ran a speech improvement service for New York actors in the 1920s and wrote detailed vocal and speech analysis in reviews of the stars of Broadway at the time (Knight, 2000).

Margaret Prendergast McLean was Tilly's assistant for a decade. She became an important speech teacher on the East Coast and her text *Good American Speech* (1928) circulated widely. McLean taught at the Leland Powers School in Boston. Edith Warman Skinner became her star pupil and then went on to study with Tilly himself in New York City between 1928 and 1933. Skinner then taught with McLean at the American Laboratory Theatre in New York City before joining the faculty at Carnegie Tech (now Carnegie Mellon). For 25 years, Skinner trained many actors and teachers and established herself as America's foremost teacher of speech. She left Carnegie Tech to teach at the Juilliard Drama Program, under the direction of John Houseman, where she continued to train a generation of American actors, including Kevin Kline and F. Murray Abraham, both at Juilliard and within the profession.

Her textbook *Speak with Distinction* was first published in the 1940s. In 1990, it was revised by Timothy Monich and Lilene Mansell and published by Applause Books. The Skinner method is taught at many major drama schools in the United States, including Carnegie Mellon School of Drama, Juilliard Drama Division, NYU's graduate program in acting, and the American Repertory Theatre at Harvard, among a number of others.

The Skinner method teaches what is termed *good American speech for the theater*, much like the Received Pronunciation taught in drama schools of Great Britain. The student is taught a modified Skinner version of phonetics as the student learns a prescriptive way of speaking. One of the method's goals is to rid students of regionalisms. Most Skinner teachers introduce the student to good American speech immediately upon entry into drama school. The teacher records the student and the student's speech patterns are analyzed and compared to those of good American speech. Specific texts such as verse and poetry rich in particular sounds are used to help the student become more adept at the good American speech dialect. They are drilled in the identification of the phonetic symbols with the appropriate sounds. The method employs many rules about speech production, use of elisions and inflections, as well as choice of words to emphasize. Some Skinner teachers use the *ask list* for many *a* sounds (a sound often used in the maritime northeastern states and provinces of North America) and delete *r* coloring in final syllables for classical text. In the past, the dialect sounded like what many refer to as mid-Atlantic, such as the dialect used by Orson Welles. Anne Bancroft (particularly in the film *The Graduate*) and Lauren Bacall use a more modern version of good American speech. Most training programs modify the sounds to sound more "American" but may teach the more "traditional" good American speech so the student has it in his repertoire (Knight, 2000).

A well-trained Skinner actor will possess a good sense of language, an ability to distinguish subtle sound differences as well as lengths of sounds, sound changes required for dialects, and verse structure. He will have confidence with classical text and "style" pieces. Because the Skinner method provides an excellent foundation in structure of sounds, structure of syntax, and numerous tools to apply in analyzing language, a Skinner-trained actor should have the ability to make technical adjustments as required. As a training method it succeeds best when balanced with some of the kinesthetic-based approaches and coming later in the training process, preferably the second rather than first year of training. Skinner herself hired Robert Parks at Carnegie Mellon because she realized that his approach provided a necessary complement to the speech training. It is difficult for an actor to free the voice and body when he is, simultaneously, learning a new dialect as well as defining and working with precise articulation. This proves particularly challenging if his own habitual dialect is one far removed from standard American or if English is not his mother tongue.

Without the balance of kinesthetic approaches, the Skinner speech work can dull the student's kinesthetic sensitivity as he becomes so focused on "how it sounds," "how he should say this," rather than on what he is communicating. The approach is often taught with a judgmental and hierarchical attitude, as if the teacher looks down on certain dialects such as a working class Texas drawl or an Appalachian dialect. The student often ends up listening and monitoring himself, creating self-consciousness rather than developing the ability to employ the words as one's weapons to pursue an intention.

Another concern with the Skinner work is an overemphasis on the phonetic transcription. Students spend hours on this aspect of the work but often remain unintelligible in their speaking. When comparing notes with other colleagues one finds the same vocal and speech difficulties prevail because of the Skinner "pitfalls." In recent years, some programs no longer utilize the Skinner approach as part of its curriculum. The UCLA graduate acting program, for example, now uses the speech work of Paul Wagar (see heading later in this chapter) as its baseline for speech curriculum. Point Park University's BFA and MFA acting programs have made a transition from Skinner-based speech work to the work of Louis Colaianni (see heading later in this chapter).

Even with psychophysical approaches taught alongside the Skinner work, it is difficult for the actor not to develop a voice that masks feelings in an effort to be pleasing, rather than a voice that reveals the depths of the actor's authentic relationship to text and emotion. Some characters may not be "pleasing" at all. If the actor's training is to sound good rather than to reveal the character's deepest needs, the actor will simply not develop the ability to tap the resources needed to play challenging characters. The more sensitive actor and often the minority actor are frequently more susceptible to being derailed by rigid speech training.

Another serious problem with the Skinner training is the emphasis on *elisions* or connected speech. The Skinner training encourages the actor to elide same sounds. For example, an actor would pronounce "dead dog" as "deadog." In theory, the second word should begin with a new thought impulse, but even with extremely experienced actors, this tends not to be the case and creates gaps in clarity. I coached *Medea* at Pittsburgh Public Theater, directed by Ted Pappas and starring Lisa Harrow. My work was with the whole company but primarily with the members of the chorus who had the extremely difficult task of speaking in unison with an underscore of original music playing continuously. The chorus members were all talented and dedicated actresses. As we moved into runs and previews, however, I found that I needed to give the same clarity notes repeatedly to two of the actresses. The actors were not able to be clear because they were eliding words. Both of them had trained extensively in the Skinner speech work. Once I diagnosed the problem, I was able to give them specific notes as to where not to elide. They incorporated the notes brilliantly and the chorus became much clearer to understand as a result. In training actors it is best to evaluate whether one elides same sounds or not, depending on the context of the scene and the clarity of the text, not simply depending on a rule. In the latter approach, actors develop flexibility. Many directors, especially British directors such as Michael Langham, who frequently directs in the Unites States and Canada, expect actors to separate same-sound consonants.

In some cases, the Skinner training is presented in such a rigid manner that when one asks an actor not to elide or change some Skinner "rule," it often causes him considerable discomfort and, in some cases, resistance. Perhaps this is due to the fact that the individuals most attracted to the Skinner method tend to enjoy a tight structure, but this sort of rigidity does not serve the actor. Often young, insecure actors want a strict right/wrong format because it provides a false sense of security.

An actor should think of any system as a set of tools rather than rules. An actor must discern what is most appropriate in a given context of a play, film, or other media. There is no "one rule fits all" method. No system can substitute for an actor's intuition and ability to analyze a text.

Over the last 15 years, speech methods have been adapted to the times. Many Skinner-trained teachers employ the book *Speak with Distinction* (Skinner, 1990) as a basis for their work while incorporating other approaches as appropriate. At the Juilliard School, Ralph Zito incorporates Alexander Technique with the speech training (Zito, 2000). Deborah Hecht, Head of Voice for the MFA Acting Program at the Tisch School of the Arts at New York University, includes vigorous movement in her approach to dialects. Nancy Benjamin, Dialect and Voice Coach at the Stratford Shakespeare Festival, frames dialect work in a cultural context that enables actors to embody the dialect more fully. She describes employing a new dialect using the lovely image of the chance to wear a scarf of a different material than one normally does, experiencing a new texture. Robin Walsh, head of the MFA Acting program at Point Park University, starts class with students singing a song in the dialect and improvising as a character who speaks the dialect. She instructs the students to pick a job they can describe, as the character, using the dialect. The class may even have a meal, appropriate to the cultural context of the accent or dialect, while employing the dialect or accent while the students discuss as they eat. Robert Haley, who also serves on the Point Park faculty, has the students write short monologues or tongue twisters using the appropriate dialect. In the above-mentioned examples, the teachers help the students develop a more kinesthetic sense and sense of ownership as the student masters an extremely technical and precise skill. Another way to engage the students is to have them teach a class on a particular dialect, including both the technical (such as sound changes, rhythm, etc.) and cultural aspects of the dialect (such as history, costume, folklore, etc.). Don Wadsworth, Professor of Voice/Speech at Carnegie Mellon's School of Drama, uses this method. These types of assignments encourage students to engage their imagination as they apply the techniques being mastered.

Paul Wagar's Text and Speech Approach

Paul Wagar, who serves on the voice/speech faculty at UCLA, has developed another way of training speech based on his early training at Webber Douglas Drama School in London, England, and with Cicely Berry while he was part of the Royal Shakespeare Company. His method is also prescriptive, introducing the students immediately to general American. He uses dictionary symbols to represent particular sounds and a simplified approach to the general American dialect, combined with rigorous and specific text work. His method encourages clear text work combined with crisp articulation and use of medial *t* in Shakespeare; that is, words like *brittle* would be pronounced with the *t* sound rather than as "briddle," as many Americans do in conversational English. He would employ *r* coloring in speaking Shakespeare; that is, words like *here*, *or*, and *power* would call for pronunciation of the final *r* sound. His students do not use the *a* of the *ask* list sound found in Edith Skinner's work except for a New England or a Nova Scotian dialect. Wagar's method is simpler than the Skinner work, with more emphasis on speaking rather than writing. It is, therefore, easier to grasp for most students. His method integrates the principles of text analysis used by Cicely Berry as outlined in her book *Voice and the Actor* (1973). His method also draws on his vast experience coaching for film and theater in Los Angeles, acting at the Royal Shakespeare Company, UK, and at the Stratford Shakespeare Festival in Canada as well as serving as artistic director for Philadelphia Area Rep Theatre, Ark Theatre (L.A.), and as Head of Voice/Speech at the University of the Arts theater program in Philadelphia. He is presently developing a workbook to train actors and teachers in this method. (P. Wagar, personal communication, May 15, 2001).

Descriptive Approaches

In the past decade, some teachers trained primarily in kinesthetically based voice have developed systems to speech training using a descriptive rather than prescriptive approach. That is, the student becomes familiar with sounds and the phonetic symbol associated with the particular sound, before the teacher makes any attempt to alter the student's own dialect. The good American speech is introduced later as a dialect once the student is already fairly familiar with phonetic symbols representing particular sounds. The student examines sound from the framework of his own dialect. This can prove useful for students whose mother tongue is not English. It can also help the minority student who may initially feel that abandoning his way of speaking is a kind of sell-out. Nonetheless, over time, an actor benefits from mastering the rather old-fashioned good American speech as a useful dialect, provided it is approached as such rather than as some sort of Holy Grail. Like the Skinner approach, these kinesthetic-based methods may be taught alongside other complementary systems.

Louis Colaianni, Claudia Anderson, and Their Phonetic Pillows

Louis Colaianni, a Linklater Designated Teacher now on faculty with Shakespeare & Company and formerly with the University of Kansas, has developed an approach to speech using phonetic pillows outlined in *The Joy of Phonetics* (1994). The teacher utilizes pillows shaped like phonetic symbols. The students use the pillows as they engage in improvisational exercises, making the sounds associated with each particular pillow. This approach is designed to assist actors to discover a tactile relationship to the symbols and sounds, in order to gain a stronger physical identification to the sounds in a playful way. Claudia Anderson is also a Linklater Designated Teacher and a voice faculty member at DePaul University in Chicago. She and Colaianni give training workshops for teachers. They have published a workbook to accompany *The Joy of Phonetics,* entitled *Bringing Speech to Life* (2003). Their approach is lively, encouraging a playful approach to sound and language, which helps the student to overcome self-consciousness.

Dudley Knight and Phil Thompson Teach the Pleasure of Language

Dudley Knight, former Vice Chair, Drama, University of California, Irvine, is a Linklater-trained teacher and Master Fitzmaurice Teacher who has also developed an approach to speech training that employs a descriptive, rather than prescriptive, training. His articles appear in the books *Vocal Vision* (2000) and *The Voice and Speech Review* (2000). He encourages experimentation of all linguistic sounds, including use of the International Phonetic Alphabet through a made-up language called "Omnish." Omnish gives the actor the opportunity to improvise, investigating speech sounds from other languages as well as English. Like *The Joy of Phonetics* (Colaianni, 1994), Knight's method emphasizes the pleasure of language as it encourages physical involvement and individual expression. The teacher introduces good American speech as a useful dialect rather than as a standard.

In the last several years, Fitzmaurice teacher Phil Thompson, Head of Acting at University of California at Irvine and president of the Voice and Speech Trainers Association (VASTA), has joined Knight and together they have conducted workshops for actors and Fitzmaurice teachers in this speech approach.

The actor trained in Knight's method should have a clear and vigorous articulation and a strong connection with his overall body, voice, and imagination.

BRITISH METHODS

In Britain, voice and speech training are more integrated. Cicely Berry, Director of Voice at the Royal Shakespeare Company and author of several seminal books (*Voice and the Actor* [1973] and *The Actor and the Text* [2000]), integrates voice and text superbly. She uses imaginative physical improvisation exercises that encourage the actor's sensitivity, connecting the release of breath with the thought impulse, thus allowing the voice to reveal the truth of the text fully and clearly. Berry has coached most of Britain's top actors and combines writing exploration with voice training. She both trained and then later taught at the Central School of Speech and Drama. Her earlier work included coaching Peter Brook's celebrated *A Midsummer Night's Dream*. She is an expert in dealing with Shakespeare and has taken the work to prisons, schools, and other countries. Deeply committed to social action, she extends the boundaries of voice to support those whose voices are rarely heard, encouraging them to speak. Her work in the ghettos of Brazil was recently featured on a special for the Public Broadcasting Service.

Cicely Berry has also conducted workshops for directors in New York City, in collaboration with Jeffrey Horowitz, Artistic Director for Theatre for a New Audience. Her work and books give actors, coaches, and directors many valuable tools to incorporate into the rehearsal process. Mr. Horowitz is of the vanguard of artistic directors who have helped raise the consciousness of the American theater community regarding the vital importance of voice and text work throughout the rehearsal process. He regularly invites Berry to coach and give workshops and hires vocal coaches on Theatre for a New Audience's productions with obvious artistic benefits. Antoni Cimolino, General Director of the Stratford Shakespeare Festival, Canada, is another forerunner in North America with his recognition of the importance of voice and Alexander work. He follows in the footsteps of earlier artistic directors Robin Phillips, David Williams, and Richard Monette, who all supported the integration of this work into rehearsal and performance within the context of a repertory company.

Another noteworthy teacher was the late Michael McCallion, author of *The Voice Book* (1998). Mr. McCallion's book is particularly useful because he incorporates the principles of the Alexander Technique in his approach and insights about the voice. Andrew Wade, formerly Head of Voice at the Royal Shakespeare Company and now vocal coach at the Guthrie Theater, and Francis Thomas, Head of Voice, Bristol Old Vic, are also teachers who combine voice, speech, and text work extremely effectively.

Patsy Rodenburg coached at the Royal Shakespeare Company under Cicely Berry and also trained at the Central School of Speech and Drama. She was formerly Head of Voice at the Royal National Theatre of Great Britain. She's authored *The Right to Speak* (1993), *The Need for Words* (1994), *The Actor Speaks* (2000), and others. Her books are filled with vital perspectives on voice and text, providing valuable information for the director and actor.

These methods succeed particularly well when combined with the Linklater or Fitzmaurice method. Both the Linklater and Fitzmaurice work deal with the psychophysical connection of breath support on a profound level and therefore offer crucial pedagogical steps in building a solid foundation in the voice and speech work.

Summary

In the final analysis, the best approach involves a balance and integration of a number of techniques. Using the best components of a variety of approaches creates less of a division between voice and speech training. Emphasis on the thought propelling the sound in whatever approach employed increases the chance of developing a fully integrated actor. This way, the inner life of the character and the intention of the character are intrinsically woven into the freedom of the voice and body. Ultimately, one hopes that the actor synthesizes internal emotional life with clarity of intention, vocal ease, and precision of speech combined with guts, support, and imagination. A director will find himself in situations collaborating with actors from many training backgrounds and some familiarity with the characteristics of these systems will make the director more adept at comprehending the actor's resume and more able to develop a specific vocabulary to assist actors. The director who understands the nuances of voice, speech, and text possesses sensitivity to the actor's journey that is invaluable in the rehearsal and performance process. This increases the chance for expressive, articulate, and supported voices to express truth and passion with clarity of thought. Actors capable of this will surely affect an audience more deeply.

CHAPTER 4

Voice and the Alexander Technique

F. M. Alexander referred to his technique as "psycho-physical re-education." One of the principles of the Alexander technique is balance and proper alignment. Alignment refers to the manner in which an actor stands and moves that allows for maximum ease and appropriate breath support. On a deeper level, the Alexander Technique not only deals with alignment but enhances the delicate interplay of the actor's thought, breath, and movement impulses. The actor needs to move with ease, finding the most flexibility without excess tension. If an actor plays Richard III, which requires uneven carriage, he must find an inner kinesthetic balance within the posture to enable the vocal relaxation necessary to deliver heightened text for 3 hours, without vocal strain. If the actor does not achieve this balance, the posture itself can create the potential for vocal tension and possible vocal damage. The incorporation of this inner balance, complementary to voice training, provides a challenging task for the actor.

In a professional rehearsal and subsequent performance of *Uncle Vanya* by Anton Chekhov directed by a talented European director, the actress playing Sonya delivered her final speech sitting at a table, collapsing her torso over it, with her neck arched forward. She produced all the sounds with little breath support and this caused her to strain to get any sound out at all. She spoke this beautiful text with a great deal of emotion and was clearly committed, but she spoke with so much vocal tension and tension in the neck muscles that it was difficult to hear and understand this poignant speech. It was also uncomfortable to listen to. This, combined with the poor alignment, caused a strangled, feeble, and monotone sound. Sadly, the director was not familiar with the Alexander work and vocal techniques. If he had been, he could have referred her to an Alexander teacher well versed in acting and voice issues who would have helped this actress find the depth of vocal expression necessary to honor the ladder of thoughts in this extraordinary text. The Alexander coach could have suggested that the actress sit up on her sitting bones and lean forward from the hip joints, thereby allowing the expanse and full circumference of the back and pelvic muscles. This would have helped her find a fuller breath support for her sound. She became caught up in forcing an overall "feeling" of the text, rather than putting her attention on the objective of the speech, using the language to clearly express the ideas. If only this actress could have focused on the thoughts propelling the sounds, instead of attempting to force the emotion and, hence, the voice, the audience would have experienced the full impact of this exquisite text.

In a student production at Carnegie Mellon, an actor was blocked to sing while lying on a bench with his head off the bench and his neck arched backwards. This position created a constriction in the neck muscles, and made it nearly impossible for the actor to gain the appropriate breath support to create an open sound. The actor strained vocally, causing a raspy sound, as his neck muscles became tighter and tighter, with the veins popping out and his face turning red. He subsequently lost his voice. A director wants to encourage movement in which the head is lined up with the rest of the spine in order to prevent this situation. Attaining proper voice usage involves changing habits. The Alexander Technique specifically addresses the thinking that causes the habits that create tension.

ALEXANDER AND THE DEVELOPMENT OF HIS TECHNIQUE

Although many people associate the technique with movement, in fact, Alexander developed his technique specifically to deal with faulty voice usage. Alexander did not use the term *mind/body* as he did not make that separation in the first place. Instead, he referred to our *use*, meaning the psychophysical relationship of thought and its impact on activity.

Frederick Mathias Alexander was born in Australia in 1869. He specialized in "recitations" of Shakespeare, but when he performed, he continually lost his voice. After he was unable to find an effective medical remedy, he spent a decade studying his movement patterns in front of a mirror. Alexander analyzed the "habits" that were causing the vocal misuse, noticing the following as he began to recite:

1. He tightened his neck muscles;
2. This caused his chin to lower;
3. This resulted in his larynx tightening and pulling down; and
4. His breath support became shallow.

He discovered that he was not able to stop these habits at will. He was able, however, to prevent pulling back his head, which resulted in the disappearance of the other two habits. As he began to master this new approach, his hoarseness stopped. He began to understand that patterns of use were not only physical but involved mental conceptions as well. He coined the idea of *inhibition* from these observations. Before he started a habitual movement, he stopped and "inhibited" the tense habit before it began. He then gave himself new thought directions related to the movement: let the neck be free, to allow the head to go slightly forward to go up, to allow the back to lengthen and widen. He named these the *means whereby* (Gelb, 1996, p. 80). Many of the principles of voice training do include the idea of inhibition or "stop" (although the voice teacher may not necessarily refer to the idea in quite the same way). Alexander found if he concentrated on the end result, his habitual tension returned. He termed this *end gaining*. If he focused on the steps to get there, however, he was able to perform the given task without the tension returning. The Alexander Technique trains the mind to bypass its initial response to specific stimuli that cause tension.

Many people think of Alexander work as "relaxation" to the point of collapse or lacking in presence. This is not an accurate understanding of the work. The Alexander Technique is an approach that helps actors (and other artists and indeed anyone in any walk of life) to find the right balance of tension required for a given vocal activity, while maintaining the maximum ease. A violin string does not produce sound if it is too loose, and if it is too tight it breaks. As with the violin string, the actor needs to find the proper *tonus* in her voice use. She needs ease to allow the full impact of the thought to express itself through the voice, with commitment and strength. If the commitment is not enough, the voice will be breathy and not carry; and if the voice is too constricted, too much pressure on the vocal folds will result in "pressing" the voice, which can injure the delicate tissue of the vocal folds. What Alexander discovered helped him find that appropriate tonus while he performed Shakespeare. He then developed his ideas further so he could communicate this practice to others.

Alexander found that he could teach others this technique by talking to an individual and simultaneously guiding the pupil with gentle touch of his hands as he tended to his own use, in the manner described above. By directing the student to develop more awareness of her habitual tensions and teaching the student how to inhibit (or stop to observe) the habitual response, the student could over time bypass these habitual tensions. He worked with actors and became known as "the breathing man." One positive by-product of freeing the head, neck, and torso relationship is more fluid and easy respiration. His article entitled "On Breathing," which appears as a chapter in *The Essential Writing of F. Mathias Alexander: The Alexander Technique* (Alexander, 1967), remains one of the clearest descriptions of the mechanics of breathing available. Alexander developed a series of ways to explore the technique called "procedures," which include the "whispered *ah*," chair work, table work, and position of mechanical advantage. Some of these are outlined at the end of the chapter, and further reading and resources about the Alexander Technique are listed in Resources at the end of the book.

At the International Congress on the F. M. Alexander Technique, held in Oxford, UK, the late Walter Carrington, who trained with F. M. Alexander himself, expressed the Alexander idea like this in his keynote speech: "We become aware of what we are doing that is causing the problem and then we do our best to prevent it" (Carrington, 2004).

The application of the Alexander Technique specifically to performance and activities began with Marjorie Barstow (1899–1995), an American who trained with F. M. Alexander in 1933 and then, in

Boston, assisted Alexander's brother A. R., whom F. M. Alexander trained in the technique. She returned to Lincoln, Nebraska, where she worked on a ranch and in this setting became interested in applying the Alexander principles to everyday activities of her life on the ranch. She also worked a great deal with performers and trained a number of Alexander teachers, including Bruce and Martha Fertman, who founded the Alexander Alliance, a teacher-training program based in Philadelphia, with sister schools in New Mexico, Germany, Japan, Korea, and Canada.

Personal Experiences with the Alexander Technique

During my Alexander teacher training, I observed Fertman working with a bassist named David Jernigan in Philadelphia. David is over 6 feet tall and rather imposing, whereas Bruce is an agile and wiry man of small frame. He almost wrapped himself around Jernigan as he guided David with hands on as Jernigan played the bass. Fertman, Jernigan, and the bass appeared to merge into one entity. As Fertman guided Jernigan, the sound of the instrument changed dramatically. The sound became richer; I perceived the notes more precisely and clearly and the overall impact of the music penetrated me in a much deeper way. While studying at Sweet Briar Residential Alexander Summer Program, I was performing a monologue I had performed many times in the context of performing my play.[1] On this particular occasion, however, Fertman guided me both verbally and through hands on and, as he did so, the character overtook me to such an extent that I really did not understand why people were laughing because I, as the character, was so intent on what I was saying that the comic irony completely escaped me. At a certain point, I had no idea whether Fertman was still working with me with his hands on or not because I was so involved with the ideas I was communicating. One of the many strengths of the Alexander Alliance training includes a generosity of spirit that Fertman brings to his teaching, a spirit that permeates the whole school in a positive manner.

---

[1]The character of Lil in *A Particular Class of Women*, by Janet M. Feindel, included in the anthology *Singular Voices*, published by Canada Playwrights Press.

A similar experience happened to me when I was assisting at the Alexander Alliance School in Germany.[2] Martha Fertman was leading the teacher trainees in a session on group teaching. She requested that I "play" one of the students. The task was to pick an activity and the designated teacher trainee would work with the student on that activity using solely the principles of the technique, that is, not giving any acting notes, music notes, and so on. I offered to work on the monologue of Charlotta, from Anton Chekhov's *The Cherry Orchard*, Act II, in German, something I had been working on just for fun for some time as I had been slowly learning German. Alexandra Buschman (graduate of Alexander Alliance, Germerode, Germany, 2008), the "teacher" trainee, began to work with me. She placed one of her hands on my sternum and the other between my shoulder blades on my back and asked me to put my attention on allowing more sense of space between her hands as her touch gently encouraged my awareness in this area. To my amazement, I became completely overtaken by the character and began to sob. One of the lines about Charlotta's parents' dying moved me in a manner it never had before. I experienced a profound sense of Charlotta's image of herself as a displaced person; and all this while I was acting in another language. Buschman did not give me any acting notes, but simply asking me to be more aware of the space between my sternum and shoulder blades allowed me to free up my overall use, which in turn enabled me to connect to the piece in a more spontaneous, deep, and imaginative way. The accepting manner—in both instances—as well as the subtle and profound technique helped me as the actor delve more into the characters.

While I was working on a character with Michael Frederick, he helped me incorporate the Alexander idea of length in the neck and freedom in the occipital joint (the joint between the neck and the skull, about at the hairline of the nape of the neck) in a manner that suited the intention of the character. He even suggested how to lengthen at a particular line in which the character was embracing her sense of authority on a specific subject. This approach gave me much more confidence and ease in playing the character.

Once in a class with Frederick I began to cry, simply because of the release of tension I experienced. He carried on with the class

---

[2]Alexander Alliance, Directors of Education, Bruce Fertman and Martha Fertman, Administrative Director Karin Boskins, Germerode, Germany, November, 2007.

in a gentle manner. I had the sense that he took in my tears but didn't make a big thing of them. I found it interesting because often in voice and acting training when an actor cries, the teacher often draws attention to it and attempts to exploit it in some manner. I commented to Frederick after our session that I found the way he dealt with my emotional release helpful and that I didn't feel judged or exploited in any way. He said, "I have Walter [Carrington] to thank for that. He always said, 'Just treat your student the same way you would treat a friend if the friend were upset. Just listen and offer support. Don't delve, and just continue with the work.'" In all the above-mentioned instances, I had already been studying and teaching the Alexander Technique for several years and these experiences only reinforced my belief in the practical, aesthetic, and affirming value of the Alexander Technique for the actor.

Benefits for the Director

When a director has a foundation in the Alexander Technique, then she can learn to block (stage) scenes in such a way that encourages balanced alignment and easy breath support. If an awkward position is unavoidable, the actor should be encouraged to think of the head away from the torso, softening the neck, and releasing (not pushing) the shoulders down as much as possible, maintaining the kinesthetic sense of the whole body. The position itself may look constricted, but the challenge of the artist is to find an inner release in a given position. The actor should be guided to search for the most efficient movement, using the least amount of tension possible. The beauty of the Alexander Technique is that, with imagination, the principles can be applied to any performance situation.

A director may want to block one actor standing talking to another actor sitting down, for example. The standing actor may tend to jut the neck forward, in a "chicken neck" fashion, cutting off her breath supply. If the standing actor needs to look up or down, she should be encouraged to do so from the occipital joint, that is, the joint at the top of the spine at the skull, rather than at the seventh vertebra, located at the back of the neck, at the same level as the collarbones. This way the actor can achieve the desired posture without creating tension in the neck area, causing undue strain on the vocal mechanism. Actors should not be blocked too close together, especially if one actor is much taller than the other. The taller actor will tend to lean forward from the neck in a way that looks awkward and prevents access to proper breath support and hence full vocal power.

Body Mapping

William and Barbara Conable developed the concept of *body mapping* in depth. Barbara Conable, who worked with Marjorie Barstow for many years, delves into her concept of body mapping in her book *How to Learn the Alexander Technique* (1995). Alexander noted that many individuals have a "debauched kinesthetic sense," and thus part of Alexander training includes addressing these misconceptions by helping an actor develop an accurate internal picture of her body in keeping with the actual skeletal and muscular structure. A ballet dancer may walk around with her feet turned out because of dancing in that position on a daily basis and yet think that the feet are parallel. When the dancer actually puts the feet in parallel, she may well have the sense that the feet are turned in or "pigeon-toed." Our heels, for example, are slightly behind, not aligned with our ankles, although shoe advertisements may give that impression. The bottom of our head is not our chin, but the roof of the mouth, as the jaw is a separate bony structure below the skull. When we wish to move the torso, the joints are at our hips, not our waist. Fashion often contributes to some of these misconceptions. Bruce Fertman would say, "The waist is a waste." The collar on a man's shirt leads us to perceive that is where the neck ends when, in fact, it ends at the collarbones.

Actors need an accurate body sense to know where they are on stage, to understand the breathing mechanism, and to know where the larynx "lives" in the body, the location of the diaphragm, and so on (see Appendix). Many vocal and yoga techniques focus on visualizing the breath in the stomach. This is fine for achieving relaxation in the abdominal muscles, which do indeed participate in the breathing process. In fact, however, we do not breathe "into our bellies"; we breathe into our lungs, and the diaphragm and intercostal muscles expand to allow us to do that. As our lungs and diaphragms expand, our abdominal muscles drop and release to allow more space for the lungs and diaphragm. (This is why one should not eat a large meal before acting or singing on stage, as the full stomach makes it more difficult for the abdominal muscles to relax.) Many actors and singers are taught to push out the diaphragm in front, just below the sternum, as if it is some kind of a pouch. This inaccurate anatomical picture creates considerable tension. This body map does not allow the actor or singer to find full support because the performer's perception does not include the full scope of the diaphragm, lungs, and intercostal muscles that surround the circumference of the whole torso. The impact of this faulty thinking is that the actor will not be heard or understood when her back is to the audience and it may increase the risk of vocal strain.

When I coached at the Stratford Festival, I worked a great deal on increasing back awareness and back resonance with the actors, and included explorations in the daily vocal warm-up that encouraged this. An actress brought in for one production was the only person on stage not working in a way that included the back awareness. The festival theater at Stratford is a thrust stage (three quarters), so someone's back will invariably be to the audience at some point. When the other actors turned away from the audience, one could still hear and understand them, but when this actress turned, because of her lack of openness in the back, her text was garbled and her voice barely audible. Because she was playing the leading female role, this clearly took away from the success of the production.

The awareness of the back is a linchpin of the Alexander work. When an actor comes on stage with three-dimensional body awareness and the voice emitting in all directions, with ease and confidence, there is nothing more exciting in a production.

An accurate body map is also enormously helpful to actors dealing with period costumes, so they can wear the costume as if it is actually clothing. When actor Robert Haley played the Emperor in *Amadeus* at the Stratford Shakespeare Festival, Canada, Desmond Healey, the costume designer, suggested the following: "This is how this guy dresses every day, just like you wear blue jeans. Don't wear the costume like you are dressed up but like it's something you throw on everyday." An accurate body map helps the actor achieve this ease because her body can move and meld with the clothes, rather than the clothes creating a constriction that reads "costume" rather than "clothing."

Alexander Technique and Training

The Alexander Technique should be incorporated in all aspects of actor and director training, and it is included in the core curriculum of most respected schools, including Juilliard, NYU, London Academy of Dramatic Art, Yale, UCLA, Folkwang Hochschule in Germany, and many other theater programs. Sessions occur individually and also with group classes. The Alexander principles can be applied to any activity or situation, and they provide a flexible and strong basis for *any* theater training program. The method deals with the interplay of self-image and movement, particularly useful for the director who needs to comprehend actor motivation and its relationship to physical actions.

Fight directors also gain enormously from studying the Alexander Technique so that they are able to integrate the principles of healthy alignment and supported voice usage into the fight choreography. The Alexander Technique can enable fight directors to encourage more back awareness and clearer understanding of body mapping. This will help actors achieve more confidence in the choreography, as they will have a better sense of where they are in space.

Another benefit of the Alexander work is that one often experiences a sense of being grounded while still feeling light, a sense of being awake and present to the moment that allows the actor to be more attuned to her environment and more responsive on stage. This is of course a great asset to the rehearsal and encourages more dynamic performance.

The student is taken through a series of "procedures" exploring "positions of maximum mechanical advantage," that is, ways we can move with the most ease and making the most efficient use of our joints. One activity involves getting in and out of a chair (often referred to as "chair work"), which we do multiple times daily, using the Alexander principle of head leading and body following as a way to practice the principle of inhibition. Teachers of the Alexander Technique also teach *constructive rest* done on the floor or on a table. Sometimes the teacher will place a book under the student's head to align the head with the spine, so the head is not falling backwards and thus causing strain in the neck. The student places the feet flat on the floor, with knees up, thinking the energy up through the knees to the ceiling and paying attention to the direction of the head away from the spine, sensing the width and length of torso. The teacher then works with the student in a hands-on fashion to guide the student kinesthetically to integrate the Alexander principles. The teacher often works with the student to release the neck and shoulder muscles through the hands, guiding the student to find more width and expanse in the muscles, thereby releasing tension. The teacher often works with lifting the leg of the student in a variety of ways, to help release tension in the hip joints. The teacher often guides the student to free tension in the back muscles and help the student gain a keener sense of her skeletal structure. The teacher needs to employ the principles in her own use and thereby communicate these to the student both verbally and kinesthetically. The student can often make more sense of the principles in a lying-down position and then apply these principles in standing activity. Even without the gift of a teacher, just lying in constructive rest for a few minutes a few times a day, thinking of directing the knees up toward the ceiling and having the thought of the head directed away from the torso, benefits the student a great deal.

Elizabeth Langford, a master Alexander teacher trained by Walter Carrington who teaches in Leuven, Belgium, told me a story about a student of hers who was a blue-collar worker, with no background in the Alexander Technique and not necessarily the most typical of students. She said he came to class and then returned a month later and he had improved considerably. She asked him what he had done and he said, "I did that constructive rest you taught me every day, as you suggested" (E. Langford, personal communication, July 2005). This is a valuable way to begin a vocal warm-up or rehearsal or just start one's day, and it works for anyone who practices it.

ALEXANDER TEACHER TRAINING

Numerous schools specializing in training the Alexander Technique exist around the world. The training takes a minimum of 3 years, as the teacher needs to fully incorporate the principles in her own use. Nonetheless, individuals who are not teachers can still employ the basic principles at the onset of study. Some teachers now work less on the procedures and focus more on applying the Alexander principles to a variety of activities. In addition to guiding the student to getting in and out of a chair and "monkey" and "table work," the teacher may also help the student apply the Alexander principles while the student is acting, singing, playing the violin, sitting at a computer, or whatever activity that student needs to contend with, as in the examples of working with acting and playing a musical instrument described earlier in the chapter. This provides a practical application to the training. Working with activities helps keep the incorporation of the technique fluid, eschewing the idea that the Alexander Technique is a "position." The Alexander Technique is a way of changing our perceptions in a manner that allows us to change habits that interfere with our fullest ease and expression.

Some traditionally trained Alexander teachers can become rigid in their approach, but this is not the goal of the Alexander Technique and this rigidity is not something Alexander himself espoused. Individuals should experience more freedom and ease after an Alexander session. Although it is natural to find something new unfamiliar, an Alexander lesson should not leave one with a sense of stiffness. If an individual experiences rigidity, then it may be best to seek out another teacher. Alexander work is delicate and rather personal, so it is important for the student to have a sense of comfort with the teacher. In many disciplines, sometimes the disciples become more fixed in their thinking than the master himself ever intended, and when this occurs, it can hinder progress in the technique.

Acting and directing students benefit enormously from this method. The most obvious benefit is that the actor frees herself of neck tension, which allows the larynx to function more effectively. The actor's breathing becomes more easeful and efficient, allowing for a more natural sound in the delivery of text. Directors obviously benefit from a basic knowledge of how alignment affects vocal production.

The idea of alignment is not new. Such disciplines as yoga, karate, tai chi, dance, and mime all emphasize alignment. Moishe Feldenkrais developed an approach to movement rather complementary to the Alexander Technique. He formulated a series of exercises designed to change movement patterns and to integrate physical and mental awareness with body movement. The Feldenkrais approach promotes more flexibility and more ease of movement by examining and altering the thought processes. The exercises generally result in more efficient breathing and increased kinesthetic awareness. The exercises blend well with vocal training methods, particularly at the beginning of the vocal warm-up.

The Alexander Technique, however, addresses more than simple alignment; it also deals with how one trains the mind to circumvent these thought processes that interfere with the freedom of movement. Alexander stressed *conscious control* of the individual. If we can learn to stop our habitual response, then we can make choices to do whatever we do in more easeful and efficient ways. The "Alexander" way of thinking encourages what Alexander refers to as more efficient "use of the self." The Alexander Technique's unique approaches to the perceptual aspects of alignment provide tools that specifically enrich voice and movement usage.

Explorations Based on Alexander Principles to Incorporate into the Rehearsal Process

A director may take cast members through the following explorations to help the actors integrate ease into their performance. It is probably best to inform actors at the onset—even in the audition process—that kinesthetic explorations will be included in the process. Some actors, understandably, can develop a cynicism to any nontraditional approaches, but if they know ahead of time and understand the purpose, they tend to respond more positively; therefore, these sorts of explorations are best introduced earlier in the process, before things get too set. Some actors have difficulty exploring new methods as they approach the previews and opening of the shows. One wants to always be sensitive to the mood of the rehearsal and adjust accordingly. Because these are explorations, there is always a certain risk involved in that one exercise may work really well at one juncture or with one particular cast and then at another time not work well at all. Sometimes one doesn't know until one attempts a particular exploration, so if something does not work, it is best not to force it but to go on to something else or wait for another time. It is useful to set the exploration up as just that, so actors do not feel as if they are auditioning or being judged in some way. This would rather defeat the purpose.

- Walk forward, and then walk backward. Notice in what part of the body the impetus for the movement comes from. Then walk forward while thinking of walking backward. Usually actors find that this allows more three-dimensional awareness of the back and side of the body, particularly around the ribs. Then repeat this sequence with text and see how this informs the text. (Inspired by Robert Parks, Professor Emeritus of Voice/Speech, School of Drama, Carnegie Mellon University.) This exploration is useful at the beginning of rehearsals, and is especially appropriate during the segment of rehearsal devoted to text work when often everyone is sitting at the table for long periods of time, to keep people lively and in their bodies.

- Lift one arm pointing up above the head and the other arm out to the side to kinesthetically think of up and wide. Use this walking and then use it again with text. Then let the movements go and notice how this has informed the text. This is particularly useful in an intense scene. Several actors can do the movement and, again, let it go and repeat the scene and see how the exercise impacts the delivery. This exploration is especially useful when rehearsing an intense scene to help the actors maintain their ease as the stakes increase. For example, one might rehearse the scene, then repeat doing this exercise without the arms, and then go back to the scene and see how this informs the approach. The actors should experience more freedom. (Inspired by Frank Ottiwell, Actor and Alexander teacher, American Conservatory Theater, San Francisco.)

- Walk around the room, imagining a second head on top of one's head. Then imagine a fancy hat on top of one's head. Look around and notice the other imaginary hats, and see how this impacts one's thought and movement. This would work best early in the rehearsals as a warm-up exploration. One could then repeat this with text, still imagining the second head and the hat. Then take the text again, without the second head and hat and see what new kinesthetic discoveries come. This works well as a warm-up technique, to loosen actors up and get them more comfortable.

- Exaggerate your habitual tension and change positions; walk around, carrying the tension. Then take a moment just to think about the head leading, allowing the neck to free; allow yourself to include the full circumference of the rib case and notice how that changes your habit. This would work best earlier in the rehearsal process before things become too set, or one might insert this when a particular scene seems stuck, to loosen people up.

- Repeat the above exercise, exaggerating tension but as you speak text. Then think of the head leading, allowing the neck to free, allowing yourself to include the full circumference of the rib case, front, side, and back, and sense how this informs your delivery as you take the text again.

- In constructive rest, lie on the floor, with a book or towel under your head. The book or towel should be high enough to support the head so it does not fall back, but not to bring the head so far forward the chin is squeezed toward the chest and pushing in on the larynx. Think of the space above the head; put your attention to the curve of the neck; think of the width across the shoulder girdle, allowing space between each shoulder blade; notice the width of the ribs and the distance between the sternum and the back ribs and spine. Notice the curve of the small of the back, the weight of the pelvic bones; kinesthetically sense (or my word, *kinesense*) the thigh bones into the kneecap, and then the calf bones below the knee, allowing a bit of space in your mind's eye between the kneecap and the knee joint; then kinesense the ankle bones and the heel slightly behind the ankle and the bones of the feet. One may also take this sequence the other way around, starting at the feet and moving upward in the constructive rest position, something I learned from Nadia Kavan in her studio in Köln, Germany.

A director could allow a few minutes at every rehearsal for constructive rest to help center the actors. This would be useful before or after the vocal warm-up. The other exercises might be woven into rehearsals as appropriate.

- Allow the breath in through the nose, lips closed with a slight smile, thinking of something pleasant. Open the mouth, let the jaw open and let the breath release on a whispered "ah." This helps wake up our awareness, open up the nasal passages, lift the soft palate, and wake up the face.

- This exercise helps actors ground themselves.
  Stand with feet hip width apart. Sense the space above and behind the head and the skull and the space between the front of the skull at the forehead and the back of the skull. Sense the weight of the skeleton while sensing the head directing away from the torso (this is not a movement but rather a thought). Sense the shoulder blades and the space between them. Picture space between the sternum and the back ribs. Sense the space from the front of the pelvis to the back of the pelvis, then the space on each side of the pelvis. Then allow the awareness of the back of the arms, the back of the legs, the ankles and the feet. Sense the soles of the feet on the floor, the sit bones dropped and the tailbone dropped as the spine moves up the torso, into the center of the skull. Just taking a few moments to stop and do a kinesthetic check like this awakens our thinking and awareness—a great tool to use before a rehearsal.

CHAPTER 5

VOX EXPLORA: What Is It?

*M*any actors and directors, particularly in the United States, take the attitude that vocal preparation before performance is only for less experienced actors. Often those with this attitude are shocked when an actor—sometimes even a very experienced actor—gets into vocal difficulties during the course of a theatrical run. While a proper vocal preparation does not prevent all vocal problems, it does prevent many vocal mishaps. Vocal preparation also facilitates a quicker recovery if and when vocal strain and/or injury do occur. Along with a solid vocal warm-up, the principles of healthy voice usage must be integrated throughout the whole rehearsal process and run. Detailed text analysis is an important component of vocal health because it is extremely difficult to speak complex text with vocal ease and support when one does not fully understand what one is saying.

I paid $75 to see a show in New York recently. The cast included a number of "name" actors, and I could tell only one had bothered to warm up before the show. It was a matinee and several of the actors' voices sounded as if the only warm-up done prior to performance was smoking a few cigarettes. The actors were inaudible, unclear in their speech, and uncommitted to the intentions of the characters. Others in the audience may not have traced it back to the actors' preparation, but I certainly heard audience members afterwards complain about the lack of commitment and clarity.

What a shame that these talented actors would not give their best to this audience!

Athletes fully accept that they must practice and prepare to perform the task at hand. Most musicians and singers do as well. No ballet dancer would attempt a *tour jeté*, a lift, or an adagio without first practicing his ballet *barre* to make sure the muscles are sufficiently toned and supple. Many actors, on the other hand, have a faulty notion that they can magically "just do it." Probably the majority of vocal misuse and injury stems from this misconception. Acting is athletic. Why would an actor do less than a dancer to prepare? Acting is the Olympics of voice use, particularly when one is acting classical text in a large theater space. The goal of a proper vocal preparation is to warm up the vocal apparatus but also to integrate the release of the voice with the actor's whole nervous system. This then enables the actor to meld with the thoughts and needs of the character in a more integrated manner. The Vox Explora is an essential tool to help reinforce this.

Vox Explora (meaning *voice exploring* in Latin) is the name I employ for the vocal warm-up I began developing over 15 years ago and continue to refine. It is a synthesis of Linklater and Fitzmaurice voice work along with the methods of Cicely Berry. I chose this name to underline the importance of integrating an imaginative component into the warm-up.

When I was first studying voice, I found practicing on my own difficult because I never knew what to focus on. My teacher at the time, David Smukler,[1] gave me the following advice: "Look for what you can discover in each exercise that is new and different from yesterday." In other words, he was suggesting I look for ways to be more "present."

Now, as a teacher, I incorporate a 5-minute meditation at the beginning of each Vox Explora to help actors quiet the busy part of the mind. The yogis call this the *manas* mind and the Buddhists sometimes refer to it as the *monkey* mind. This part of the mind is also sometimes referred to as the "critic" or the "committee" and can become extremely distracting and even destructive for an actor. "Will they like me?" "Are the reviewers out there?" "Is this my best performance?" "What will the director or other actors think?" "My

---

[1] David Smukler, Head of Voice, Theatre Department, York University, Toronto, Ontario, Canada, 1989.

costume feels uncomfortable." "Why doesn't so-and-so perform in this way?" and so on. The actor needs a way to bypass all this side chatter and gently put his attention back on his partner on stage and the task at hand. One needs to balance the monkey mind so that it does not ride roughshod over the other parts of the psyche. When one can quiet this part of the mind, it encourages our psychophysical intelligence to come more into play. By this I refer to a more primitive, expressive, and intuitive part of the mind within the body, a visceral or — if you will — more "gut" relationship to sound and language.

The most important component of the warm-up is developing more awareness of the flow of breath, without placing any imposition on it. Lynette Francis, a wonderful movement teacher at the Bristol Old Vic School in the United Kingdom and formerly of the Shaw Festival, puts it beautifully: "Think of the breath as a friend who comes to visit, someone you don't need to fuss about and that you just say 'Here is the key, there's where you are sleeping. Now look after yourself.'"[2] In other words, one wants only to observe the incoming breath and the outgoing release, not try to control it. One notices that there is a moment of waiting after the outgoing breath, the moment in which we get in touch with our desire to breathe, our impulse to speak, before we allow the breath back into us on the intake. The French verb for inhale is *inspirer*—think of the English word *inspiration*. When one is inspiring the breath, in acting terms, one is inspiring to communicate.

People sometimes approach breathing with great muscular effort, attempting to control intake and outtake. Many actors feel it is necessary to "breathe in" and then "breathe out" with a great act of will. Unfortunately, this effort, even with the best of intentions, creates more tension, which tightens muscles affecting voice production, causing a forced sound, and so is counterproductive. Or an actor pushes out the front part of the diaphragm below the sternum, as if it is a pouch, which again only creates more unwanted vocal tension. All these acts of effort only compound any existing respiratory difficulties. F. M. Alexander articulates this beautifully in his article "About Breathing" in *The Alexander Technique: The Essential Writings of F. Mathias Alexander* (Maisel, ed., 1995). (Please also see Chapter 4, Voice and the Alexander Technique.)

---

[2]Movement warm-ups at the Shaw Festival, Niagara-on-the-Lake, Canada, 1989.

One wants to develop the ability to observe the breath and increase the flexibility and stamina of the intercostal muscles. Some methods encourage actors to hold the breath for several counts after the intake. This reinforces a habit that we do not want on stage. There is a natural orchestration that happens between two characters that has to be allowed to take its own life and rhythm. An actor needs to respond spontaneously to each idea on the breath. If the actor develops the habit of holding the breath after each intake, then he interferes with the natural ebb and flow of communication that occurs on stage.

Beyond the breath awareness, the Vox Explora helps the actor fine-tune the psychophysical connection. Each sound uttered delves deeper into the actor's psyche and imagination as the muscular and nervous systems respond at a primitive level. We are training the respiratory system to respond to the thought impulse and shape the sounds with precision with the articulatory muscles in order to communicate and affect another person. This delicate interplay of responses must be integrated into all aspects of the voice preparation, and the actor must integrate this work so a fully engaged actor walks on stage. As discussed in Chapter 2 and Chapter 3, warm-ups in which the actor does vocal "exercises" without attention to physical or psychological awareness—with no focus on thought and imagination—do little to reinforce a well-balanced, full-bodied attunement in the actor. On the contrary, this sort of warm-up only serves to disconnect the actor from his deeper expression. A dancer can perform a ballet *barre* thinking only of the various muscular components ("Now I point my toe, now I lift my leg, my arm is now in second position"). Or the dancer can utilize the warm-up to stimulate and strengthen the various muscle groups and their interrelationship, while at the same time fully internalizing the rhythm and phrasing of the music, expanding the three-dimensional awareness of the body and "dancing" each part of the *barre*. By treating the *barre* like a piece of choreography in which the whole body and psyche engage fully, the dancer prepares the whole psychophysical system to respond in a more expressive manner. When the dancer activates the inner workings of the artist before she goes on stage, this frees the dancer to dance with more dynamism and nuance.

B. K. S. Iyengar (2005) describes yoga practice in the following way:

The goal of all asana practice is doing them from the core of your being and extending out dynamically through the periphery of your body. As you stretch, the periphery relates messages back to the core. From head to heels, you must find your center, and from this center you must extend and expand longitudinally and latitudinally. If extension is from the intelligence of the brain, expansion is from the intelligence of the heart. While doing the asana, both the intellectual intelligence and the emotional intelligence have to meet and work together. Extension and expansion always stay firmly rooted in one's center. They originate from the core of one's being. (p. 33)

An actor should originate the voice work from the core of his being as well. One needs an awareness of the space combined with the integration of the thought, breath, and intention. The proper preparation increases the actor's confidence and allows the actor to respond spontaneously during performance. This immediacy is what separates the great artist from the actor who delivers only a workmanlike performance.

An audience may not even consciously realize why one performance affects them more deeply than another. They may not know that the preparation of the actor made an impact on their experience, but they will definitely distinguish one performance or production as more fully satisfying over another and whether or not they can hear and understand the actors clearly. Why would any talented actor want to bring less than his full dynamic self into the performance so as to affect the audience as deeply as possible? My wonderful colleague, Alexander teacher Zoana Gepner-Mueller, puts it beautifully: "*Ganzer Körper, Ganzes Selbst*" (the German for "Full body, full self").[3]

Some actors think it may be important to warm up for stage but not for film or voice-over. I worked with a gifted actor, with a rich and beautiful voice, who had lost his voice recording a voice-over. He taped this during the morning while rehearsing a major part off Broadway in the afternoon and arrived for the afternoon rehearsal hoarse, admitting he had not warmed up vocally before recording. Fortunately, there were some Linklater remedies I was

---

[3]Conversations with Gepner-Mueller while working with Alexander Alliance Teacher Training Program, Germerode and Krefeld, Germany, 2004, 2005.

able to guide him through to help him regain his voice enough so he could still carry on through rehearsal, though not at full capacity. Of course, any vocal difficulty causes the actor and the theater management concern and stress, and in some cases, this stress can compound the vocal problem. Moral of the story: take care of your voice and vocally warm up before the voice-over, especially when one is also rehearsing a play.

In some cases, film situations challenge the actor vocally even more than stage. The actor may have to repeat an intense scene with less than ideal conditions, such as in the torrent of a river, wet and cold at some ungodly hour like 5:00 AM. Preparing vocally before such strenuous filming conditions can help prevent vocal injury and keep the actor psychologically focused so such conditions do not distract him.

Directors (as well as acting teachers and vocal coaches) cannot emphasize the importance of the vocal warm-up enough. The director cannot only reinforce the importance of the vocal warm-up but can help the actor enormously by allotting time for it within the rehearsal. Ideally during a run, the actors should have access to the stage before each performance. Directors and stage managers can reinforce this. Sound and lighting cues should not be tested during the vocal warm-up, as this is distracting to the actors. If the stage is not available and actors have to warm up in a different space, they need at least a few minutes before performance on stage so that they have the chance to adjust to the vocal requirements of the theater. The first words of the performance should not be the first words that actor has uttered on the stage that day. At the Royal Shakespeare Company in England, the whole company warms up together, from apprentice to major star (such as Ian McKellen) and the benefits are obvious.

An important part of the vocal warm-up involves warming the nervous system so articulators (lips, tongue, and jaw) respond to thought with clarity and precision, as discussed in Chapter 3, Overview of Speech Methods. I have listened to actors doing articulation exercises like robots, with little thought, less breath support, tight jaws, and a great deal of tension through the body, thinking they are doing a marvelous job of vocal preparation. Yet I cannot understand a word they are saying. It is important that when the actor practices the articulation segment of the warm-up, he incorporates the principles of healthy, effective voice usage. The actor must continue to stay connected to the thought and the breath support, keeping the tongue root and the jaw as released as possible. While most vocal warm-ups include articulation toward the end, one can experiment successfully with including articulation earlier in the warm-up in order to effectively incorporate ease and breath support, especially when doing an articulation-heavy show such as a Restoration play or the plays of George Bernard Shaw. While tongue twisters are fun (indeed, I have included a number in this chapter), one must keep the imagination engaged as one does them. It is helpful to do them as if they are little scenarios. For example, one says, "Betty bit a bit of butter, but it was a bitter bite, but a better bit of butter, Betty never bit," as if one disapproves of Betty, or as if one is a psychoanalyst attempting to analyze Betty's actions that seem odd. In other words, one must keep "the thought propelling the sound." If one is repeating by rote and not thinking, then one is training the nervous system to perform that way on stage. One must always remember that the purpose of voice training is to connect the breath and thought impulse through clear text on an open, authentic sound. It is most effective to use text that is lively, inspiring, and interesting for articulation work such as Nelson Mandela's inauguration speech (written by Marianne Williamson, *Return to Love* [Harper Collins, 1992, pp. 190–191]), Sojourner Truth's "Ain't I a Woman?" (1851), and the speeches of Dr. Martin Luther King, Jr. If a piece of text becomes stale, one should move on to something else, such as a poem or speech that feels meaningful to the actor.

A director with minimal background in voice work can lead the following Vox Explora, provided that he emphasizes that the actors maintain ease throughout. The goal is not a loud sound but a released sound, with no tension in the throat, neck, and shoulder areas. A director should be strongly encouraged, however, to study voice and speech weekly for at least 9 months; of course, if the director can study voice and speech on a regular basis for several years, this is even better. The director should remind actors of release at all times. An actor should not push from the throat for a loud sound in a warm-up, as this can tire the voice rather than prepare it properly. A gentle warm-up but fully on voice that is not breathy strengthens the voice and gives it longevity. Actors should think of release and ease in a warm-up. The Canadian opera star

John Vickers, Companion of the Order of Canada, attributed the longevity of his international career to a regular and gentle vocal warm-up.[4] The same principle applies to actors. One cannot underscore this enough.

Every warm-up should include at least a little of each of the following:

- Meditation or relaxation to quiet the mind
- Focus on the awareness of the breath without imposition
- Physical stretches designed to open up physical and mental awareness
- Gentle touch of sound
- Gentle humming
- Gentle exploration of pitches
- Stretching the intercostal muscles
- Opening of resonators, particularly in the face
- Inviting the back awareness with sound by thinking the sound releasing out the back
- Waking up the articulation muscles and incorporating this with text
- Recentering

For many years I have presented at the Care of the Professional Voice symposium in Philadelphia and one of the advantages has been listening to the talks of Dr. Robert Sataloff, an internationally recognized neurolaryngologist and ear, nose, and throat specialist who specializes in professional voice users. He is a trained classical singer, musician, and conductor as well. Dr. Sataloff stresses the importance of the "vocal cool-down" after vocal use to help prevent vocal injury when a performance is particularly strenuous vocally. He also encourages voice and singing teachers to warm up before teaching and cool down after teaching.

---

[4]Conversation with William Vickers (John Vickers' son), Acting Company member at Shaw Festival, Niagara-on-the-Lake, Canada, 1990.

The vocal cool-down should include the following:

- Centering of the mind and breath awareness
- Gentle touch of sound or humming
- Massaging the tongue root
- Relaxation of the whole body

STANDING VOX EXPLORA, #1

The Sound Quilt

This is a simple warm-up that can be led and done with beginners to advanced performers. The main thing to emphasize is release and ease, never forcing from the throat.

- Start in constructive rest. Lie on floor, feet flat on floor, knees up toward the ceiling, probably with a book under the head. Think of the energy of the knees going toward the ceiling and the energy of the head moving away from the torso, back lengthening and widening, awareness of side ribs.
- Observe the breath; think of "allowing" the breath in and then letting it release out. Notice the moment before you allow the breath back in. It is a moment of pause, of getting in touch with your need to breathe and with the text, your need to speak. You might think of the incoming breath as your connection with humanity and the outgoing breath as your contributing yourself to the world.
- Imagine the inside of the intercostals as if one were looking from inside the sternum; notice how this gives more space.
- Start with a gentle hum, just slightly higher than your habitual speaking pitch.
- *Kinesense* (kinesthetically sense) with your hands the vibrations on cheeks, top of head, throat, back of neck, and chest.

- Gently experiment with hum on different pitches; start in midrange and then as one feels more warmed up, move to higher and lower differentials in pitches.
- Move and stretch with the release of sounds.
- Gradually come to standing, keeping the neck and shoulders free by rolling over onto one side and coming up to sitting by rolling through the spine, head coming up last and coming up to standing with grace and elegance.
- Imagine coaxing sound from top of head, back of head, back of neck, face, throat, chest, back, pelvis, thighs, calves, feet, and so on, as you do a gentle pulling motion, as if the sound is taffy.
- Continue to begin the sound on a hum, on different pitches, but each time go from the hum to a vowel of choice; continue to pull the sound, imagining it like taffy.
- In a circle, imagine a "sound clothesline" across the circle. Everyone continues to hum onto different vowels and different pitches. One person releases his sound, gently pulling it from the face, for example, and another person catches the sound across the circle and then moves to a different body part, perhaps this time pulling the sound from the pelvis.
- Then imagine a "sound quilt" that everyone is holding and waving out in the sun, and the scope of the wave gets bigger and bigger and then smaller and smaller, and let the group's sound respond in kind.
- Finally, go back to just a hum, each person imagining it circulating through the whole body, and then the group can come closer and let the sound vibration move through each person.
- Each actor picks a line of text that is a bit of a mouthful and has everyone do it as a tongue twister.
- Take some inspirational text, such as Nelson Mandela's inauguration speech (Williamson, 1992) or a speech of

Dr. Martin Luther King, Jr. Read it as a group, and then have each person read it one line at a time, then one word at a time, making sure the through line of the text continues. (You can also incorporate some of the text exercises outlined in Chapter 7, Voice and Text Explorations, as well as those of the Cicely Berry text outlined in her invaluable book *The Actor and His Text*, see References.)

■ Take a moment, quiet the mind, touch sound on "huh," and at the same time include in your awareness the sense of the width of the back, the space above the head, space to the sides, space behind.

Et voila!

Alternate Vox Explora

■ Standing, one leg slightly in front of the other, cross arms across chest, go over halfway, bending from the hips; take three silent breaths in through the nose; come up on a hiss, thinking of the sound like a stream of light; then repeat on this releasing on a voiced hiss that is a *z* sound. (This exercise inspired by Patsy Rodenburg.)

■ Stretch ribs over to the right side, keeping the shoulders relaxed; wake up side ribs by massaging the intercostal muscles as far up toward underarms as possible. Come back up to center on *f-f-f*, and then reverse sides and come up on *v-v-v*.

■ *Sha/sh* exercise: Stand hip-width apart, arms up on an intake of breath; as the arms are brought down to sides, release breath on *sh*. Repeat this three times; the third time drop over on *sha* and then uncurl through the spine coming up on *sh, sh, sh, sh, sh, sh* until you are back to standing. This can be done quite vigorously as long as the throat stays free. This is a particularly good exercise to energize if one is tired. (Inspired by Francis Thomas, Head of Voice/Speech, Bristol Old Vic Drama School, United Kingdom.)

- Shake out arms, legs, and buttocks on an easy baby sigh.
- Circle head, thinking of a pencil at the end of the nose, from occipital bone and gently hum, sensing the hum in the face.
- Imagine a bunch of mosquitoes on your face and you can't use your hand to get them off. (Inspired by Liz Smith, formerly Head of Voice/Speech at Juilliard School, Drama Division.)
- Warm hands and massage jaw hinge in small circles toward nose.
- Massage tongue root, underneath chin, careful not to put pressure on larynx. Gently massage neck on either side of the larynx and back of neck, and then sternum, diaphragm, and belly. Gently hum at the same time and see if it is possible to sense the sound vibrations moving through each different area.
- Imagine touching sound on *huh* but don't actually speak; observe what happens to you physically; and then with the same ease, repeat the movement but this time with sound. This is particularly helpful when you are very tense and need to go back to the basic touch of sound without pushing.
- Touch sound, on *huh*, down from middle C for women, an octave lower for men, 3 pitches, B, B flat, A, and then back up to C, then up to G, then back down to C; then speak on *huh*. Then repeat this sequence on *huhumuh*.
- Loosen lips, blow through *brumuh*. Also do this on pitches, from E to A above middle C for women, and an octave lower for men.

Alternate Vox Explora #2: Lying Down

- Gently hum, allowing voice to warm up gradually.
- Then go from hum to *muh*; repeat a hum on *n*, and then go onto a *nuh*.

VOX EXPLORA: WHAT IS IT? 73

- Continue sound and roll over into a fetal position, then onto all fours, and then up to standing by uncurling through the spine.

- Explore different pitches on a hum; take a breath when you need to; imagine pulling sound out of different parts of body; then hum onto a vowel of choice, again exploring different pitches. Keep this going for 5 to 10 minutes. *Note*: This exercise can also be done with the actors back to back, swaying and moving the body as the actors' voices release. This also helps the actors sense the awareness of the sound resonating in the back.

- Remember to feel the hum buzzing in the lips and be aware of the area between the teeth and lips to help bring sound forward without pushing it.

- Tongue rolls (tip of the tongue behind the lower front teeth), and release on *huh*, then roll tongue forward on *yuh* (so it's *huhyuh*). Pitches are E to about B (above mid-C for women, an octave lower for men).

- *Hee* into sinus, *very gently*; really stress the sound coming "up and over the shelf," which is visualizing the sound like a conveyor belt, starting at the sacrum and lower back ribs and coming up along the spine and back of neck, releasing up and over the bone of the hard palate, through the area just below the cheek bones; pitches E to B (don't go too high on this).

- *Mee hay ah o oo*, very gently, imagining the sound vibrations out the face (if short of time, do this instead of *hee*, but it's best if both are done).

- Hum down the face as if there is a waterfall down your face.

- Rib stretch: Elbows up, wrists below elbows, stretch the front part of the ribs three times; drop elbows, wrists, and fingers. Repeat sequence, stretching the back part of the ribs, with special attention to the lower back ribs; think of ribs going down and back, and then release the elbows and arms again. Lift the elbows up, wrists below the elbows; stretch the lower front ribs and keep them expanded and then stretch the lower back ribs and keep them expanded. Then lift the shoulders and arms, as you walk the ribs up. Then drop the shoulders and arms but keep the ribs expanded and think what kind of artist you are and then say, "Absolutely fabulous!" Then release the ribs, but continue to sense the circumference and repeat the line. One can also do this with text, saying it first with the ribs expanded and then with them released while still sensing the full three-dimensionality of the torso. (This exercise is repeated in the Linklater-inspired warm-up.)

- In partners, one person rolls down through spine, releasing on *huh* as the other gently pounds on either side of spine to help loosen sound and wake up the awareness of the back. (It is important not to put pressure right on the spine itself; only on the muscles on either side of the spine.)

- Sigh sound out back; lift arms like angel wings. It helps to keep back open on *huh, hah, hey*.

- Keeping breath centered, with ease, release on the sound *hey* and image the sound in the hips, like a sound tutu, or *hey baby* in mid-range (again, around mid-C for women, low C for men); take the pitch down a few pitches, and then back up to about F–G.

- Recenter and release on *huh*.

- Drop through spine, blowing through lips; start low and then go up in pitch as you drop over. As you come up through the spine, go down in pitch; in other words, make the movement direction opposite to the pitch direction so as to keep the voice releasing.

- Articulate stressing breath and full lips, finding sensuality of consonants.

- *Be be be, bay bay bay, bah bah bah, bo, bo, boo boo boo*, then repeat same sequence on different consonants: *m, n, s, z, d, l, t, v, w, m, p*. Really use lips. You can

- massage tongue root so one is not driving the sound from the tongue; rather, think the sound up and over the hard palate.
- Then do a few tongue twisters. Choose two to three from the list, but make sure you give each one a little intention of some kind or, better yet, write your own tongue twister or some text.
- Recenter, grounding the feet hip-width apart; sense the space behind, sense the space in front, to the sides, above the head, sense the soles of the feet on the ground, back of the legs, back of the pelvis, back of the back, and back of the head, including the space between the forehead and the back of the skull. Allow space between the back teeth.

Note: Don't get too panicked if you miss something on a particular day; just try to do a little in each area. The main thing is that the warm-up is most effective when it is really gentle.

Alternate Vox Explora, #3

- Start by massaging jaw hinge, loosening sternum and diaphragm.
- Circle shoulders easily, as if you are trying to get a sweater off your shoulders.
- Gently hum as you make a head circle by imagining you have a pencil at the end of your nose.
- Stretch over to the side, hips square. Massage side ribs; come back to center releasing on an *f*. Repeat on other side, releasing on a *v*.
- Roll the head by imagining a pencil at the end of the nose and drawing a circle with it; reverse directions—the circle is coming from the occipital area.
- Hum gently, sensing the buzz on the lips as you continue to circle the head.

- Alternate humming on *ng* (or humming on an *n* is fun too), then opening up on the vowel: *ng, nga, n, na*, and *m, ma*.
- Speak *huh*—thinking of breath/sound releasing simultaneously.
- Repeat on *huhumuh*.
- *Brumuh*.
- Place tip of the tongue behind the lower teeth; hum with lips together on *m-m*, and then let the jaw release on *hey* so the final sound is *meehey*, releasing the jaw and thinking of the sound coming up and over the hard palate.
- Rib stretches: Float elbows up, stretch ribs forward, release; stretch lower back ribs, release, and drop arms.
- Clasp the hands in front and stretch the arms forward to stretch back ribs.
- Clasp the hands behind the back and lift the arms to stretch the front ribs.
- With partners: Partner A places hands on partner B's lower side ribs, and then B sighs out on sound into partner A's hands on *hey*. Keep the sound gentle; imagine it is a healing balm, as if the partner has arthritis and the sound will soothe the discomfort.
- Purse lips and release on the sound *yee* (Lessac-inspired exercise). This can also be done in a squat.
- *Z* on range: Start high and then go through range, ending on the lower notes.
- Blow through lips on range; roll through spine as one goes up in range and come up through spine as one descends in range. This opposition keeps the experience organic.
- Gentle articulation: *bee, bee, bee; bay, bay, bay; ba, ba, ba; boo, boo, boo*; repeat with *p, w, v, f, d, l, t, n, g, k, ng, dg* as in *judge* or *range*.

- Tongue twisters (see end of warm-up). This is also a good place to include text/voice explorations found in Chapter 7, Voice and Text Explorations.
- Recenter; touch sound on *huh*.
- Partner, roll down, and massage.
- Baby sigh on *huh*.

LINKLATER-INSPIRED VOX EXPLORA #3

The following vocal preparation is inspired by the work of Kristin Linklater with my additions. Most of the additions include suggested motivations to stimulate the actor's need to communicate through sound and language. The Vox Explora includes all the Linklater resonators. The resonators are explained in more detail in Chapter 6, Resonex. This particular warm-up takes about 45 minutes and requires specific training in this method. Readers should also familiarize themselves with *Freeing the Natural Voice* by Kristin Linklater (1976, revised 2007) and study with a Linklater-designated voice teacher. See Resources for more information.

Vox Explora

Lying on the Floor

Relaxation (Hollow Body). Imagine each part of the body hollow. Visualize the breath into each area: imagine the breath into the right leg, left leg, and so on. Then imagine sound into each area; picture the breath going into the body from the top of the head down through the toes; and then imagine the breath coming in through the pores of the skin, like mesh material, and releasing out through the pores; repeat with sound; become a breathing amoeba.

Purpose: To center breath, relax muscles, allow sound to release effortlessly, connect to the imagination.

Feldenkrais. In yoga corpse pose, palms of hands toward ceiling, move head to right as you move the left leg turned out along floor;

bring head and leg to center, knee toward ceiling, foot on the floor; repeat on the other side so both knees are toward ceiling.

Purpose: A gentle twist of the spine, a way to bring knees up without straining back.

Touch Sound. Touch sound on *huhuh*. Mid-C for women, lower C for men down 3 to 4 notes, including back keys, then back to C to F or G, back down to C; speak it.

Purpose: To connect to sound in an internal, relaxed way, allowing the breath and sound to release simultaneously.

Repeat sequence on *huhumuh*.

Purpose: To gently bring internal sound forward onto lips, allowing lip area to resonate, sharing the sound out, without strain.

Diagonal Stretch. Kinesense the expanse of the ribs. Bring right thigh to chest, and then left, knees bent; drop knees over to right side, look left, stretching out left arm; take right arm across to intercostals.

Purpose: Opens up rib awareness, intercostal muscle awareness; allows breath to connect more deeply.

Side Rib Stretch. Go over onto right side in a fetal type position. Place right arm under head, making sure spine is straight. Knees should be bent enough to allow lower back to round ever so slightly. Place left hand on lower left side ribs. Expand left side rib up to ceiling, then release on a hiss, then on a z. As you do this, continue to expand the ribs up toward the ceiling and notice how you can kinesense the diaphragm muscle moving up and under the ribs. Bring knees to chest, rounding small of back; repeat sequence to the left side, releasing on an f and then a v.

After you have done the above on both sides, go over into the prayer position. Stretch forward, then stretch the arms to the right, as you stretch the left side ribs, and then come back to center and stretch the arms to the left, as you stretch the right side ribs.

Purpose: Releases back after the diagonal stretch, and increases flexibility of the intercostal muscles and awareness of the movement of the diaphragm.

Coming Up to Standing

Squat onto all fours, and then bring right foot to right hand, left foot to left hand, into squat, thinking of the sitting bones up toward the ceiling, knees slightly bent, and then uncurl through the spine, head coming up last.

Purpose: To help relax abdominal muscles and let breath connection be even deeper; to relax muscles on either side of spine; to help develop awareness of spine and alignment. (*Reminder*: Keep sense of upward motion in hips; don't tuck hips under; think of lifting the pelvis through the uncurling to avoid "sitting" into the hips; keep knees soft.)

Standing Up

Blow through Lips. On *brumuh* D-G back to D (just above mid-C for women; an octave lower for men).

Purpose: Relaxes lip muscles for later articulation. (*Reminder*: Bring sound forward, keeping breath connected. If one tenses, the lips won't move, so it is a good barometer.)

Jaw Release. On *meehey* place tongue tip behind lower teeth; start with *mee* and then open jaw on *hey* but think of joining the two sounds together on *meehey*. Jaw should release back, slightly down.

Purpose: Relaxes jaw hinge muscles; can help stimulate production of saliva.[5]

Soft Palate Stretch. On *hunguh*, D-A back to D, and then speak it. Release on *huh*, then bring soft palate down to back of tongue on *ng*, making sure soft palate comes more forward than back, and then lift soft palate on *uh*. Make sure the sound is not swallowed.

Purpose: To increase flexibility of soft palate, feel space in throat, allow sound forward with ease, and be playful with the sound, connecting a full sound incorporating back ribs.

Tongue Stretch. *Huhyuh*: Sigh out on *huh* and then stretch tongue out, with tip of tongue behind lower teeth, and then release tongue back into relaxed position; repeat pitch sequence.

Purpose: To release tongue root, to stretch middle of tongue, to isolate tongue muscles from jaw movement, to think of sound vibrations moving forward even as tongue returns to neutral position.

---

[5]This exercise inspired by the late Maria Corvin, actress and voice teacher, who trained with Iris Warren and taught at George Brown College in Toronto, Ontario, Canada.

Tongue Roll. *Huhyuh, yuh, yuh*: Sigh out on sound on *huh*, then move front of tongue, with tip behind lower teeth; keep easy, relaxed, keep breath dropping, and don't push for sound.

Purpose: To increase flexibility of front of tongue for articulation, to be able to do fine movements without tightening jaw or tongue root, while keeping breath relaxed; useful for training for crisp texts such as Restoration, farce, British comedies, and so on.

Reverse Tongue Roll. *Heeyuh, yuh, yuh*: Starting with tongue tip behind lower teeth, begin with it rolled forward, then sigh out on neutral sound *huh* but it will come out *hee*; then roll tongue forward and back, a smaller movement than tongue stretch. As you get more comfortable, you can do *heehuyuyuyuluh-luh-luh-muh, muh, muh, muh.*

Purpose: To bring sound more forward, in preparation of teeth resonator; to loosen the tongue muscles and find ease in isolating the tongue, keeping jaw relaxed.

Rib Stretch. Float elbows up, wrists below elbows; stretch front ribs three times, and drop the elbows. Lift the elbows up again, then stretch the back ribs three times, release, and drop the elbows; float the elbows up again, stretch front ribs, then back ribs, then walk ribs up; keep ribs expanded, allowing the shoulders to lift; then drop arms and shoulders. Keeping ribs expanded and lifted, say a line of text or "absolutely fabulous"; then release them again, feeling ease of expansion; without holding, try to support fully, not forcing the sound from the throat.

Purpose: To feel expanse of ribs, to know where they are, and to connect to the power of the back.

Resonating Ladder

(Also see Chapter 6 on Resonex.)

Chest/Back Resonator. Praying to gods on *hah*: Arms stretch up to heavens, knees soft, release on *hah*, with head tilted back from the occipital area; keeping the neck long, start at mid-C and then work down to lower range. Don't sustain too long here; keep it easy, and then try a couple of sustained *hah*s. Make sure you support, keep the sound motivated, and ask the gods for something you want.

Purpose: To feel back/chest resonance without pushing from throat; ease and power; connection to back ribs and full body sound.

Mouth Resonator. Then back to the mouth resonator on "*huh*" mouth resonator. Feel sound bouncing off hard palate.

Purpose: To feel size of mouth; feel sound cleaning in mouth, without swallowing the sound to the back of the throat (another option is to start with the mouth resonator). For some individuals, it is easier to start with the mouth resonator, which is more in the mid-range, and then go to the chest/back.

Teeth Resonator. On *hee-hee-hee,* head forward, feel sound moving through teeth.

Purpose: To wake up teeth resonators

Hey. Then join three sounds on *hey*: try a few triads, *hey baby*, *hey mama* on different pitches, keeping the connection of the ribs and sense of an open back, and so on.

Ybuzz. Purse lips on *yee-yee-yee*; also variation, *oowee-oowee-oowee-oowee*, exaggerating pursing of the lips on the *oo*, and then smiling the lips on the *wee*.

Purpose: To feel sound in alveolar and "moustache" area; get the sound forward; particularly good for warming up the mask and preparing for British and European dialects.

Sinus Resonator: *Hee*. Purpose: To feel vibrations in sinus area, a vulnerable open area for actors.

Nasal. *Mee-mey-mah-mo-moo*, at first extremely gently, and then one can ping the sound with more intensity, provided that attention is paid to proper breath support and maintaining an open, relaxed throat.

Purpose: To wake up nasal resonance; to be more aware of using soft palate, going from a nasal sound to a non-nasal sound, keeping throat open; helps achieve greater awareness and flexibility. Nasal can be especially useful in certain kinds of character voices, dialects, and the like, but one should not be stuck in it. Again, one must approach warming up the nasal area gently so as not to cause vocal strain.

Snasal Resonator. Combine the nasal and sinus on *mee-mee-mee-may-may-may-my-my-my*, thinking of the sound starting at the bridge of the nose and moving across the sinus area below the cheekbones and then circling into the sinus area above the eyebrows. One must take special care to keep one's support as it is easy to strain in this resonator. If one is experiencing vocal fatigue or coming down with a sickness, it is best to avoid this resonator until one is stronger.

Head. *Kee:* Thinking sound out of the skull, again making sure to maintain proper breath support.
 Purpose: Head resonance; build eventually for scream if necessary.

Range. Blowing through lips, high to low, low to high range on *brumuhmuhmuh*.
 Purpose: Find ease of range, incorporate all that has proceeded.

Articulation. (See list of tongue twisters at end of chapter for alternate articulation exercises.)
 Consonant sequences:

- *Be, bay ba*, etc.
- *Bee, bee, bee; bay, bay, bay; ba, ba, ba*
- *Pee, pee, pee; pay, pay, pay; pa, pa, pa*

Repeat with *vee, wee, lee, nee, dee, tee, gee, kee, she, jdee* (as in the beginning and final consonant sound of *judge*).
 Purpose: To exercise muscles of articulation, maintaining breath support and ease.

Tongue Twisters. It is important here to keep relaxed and incorporate breath support and all areas that have been opened up. Then move on to tongue twisters, making sure that the breath support and thought remain easy and the imagination is engaged. It can be useful to give actors intentions to play with; for example with the tongue twister "The girl stood on the balustrade balcony, inexplicably mimicking him, hiccuping, and amicably welcoming him in," one can say it as if one is telling a tale of gossip, acting as a detective, or as if one is a psychoanalyst analyzing why the girl is doing this.

You can also write your own tongue twisters or ask the cast to write ones suited to a particular show. Another effective method is to ask each actor to pick a line of text he finds particularly challenging and the whole cast repeats it. By teaching it to the cast, the actor has to deal with whatever the hurdle is that makes it a challenging line to deliver. (See end of section for selection of tongue twisters.)

Purpose: To move articulation muscles, connecting with thought in more complex patterns.

Back to touch of sound on *huh* to make sure you are still centered.

Purpose: To reinforce ease in the breath support.

Text. Now it's fun to try some text, experimenting with pitch, range, and resonators, and then let it go and don't impose; see what you find, dance the text, move, swing.

Purpose: To make sure the principles of voice usage are applied to text with physical ease.

After warming up articulators, make sure to keep jaw relaxed and breath easy. Do some kind of relaxation afterward.

Enjoy your vocal expression!

SELECTION OF TONGUE TWISTERS FROM VARIOUS SOURCES

The wild wolf roams the wintry wastes.

Six sick sad sparrows sang stupid songs.

Now nine naughty, nice nurses need nifty necklaces.

The trend of the times was tiresome, tedious, and tame.

The lone lustful lovers lounged in the lane.

Wonderful wild women.

Many magnificent men.

Betty bit a bit of butter but it was a bitter bite but a better bit of butter Betty never bit.

A pale pink proud peacock pompously preened its pretty plumage.

Lovely Lulu loved lazy Leonard but he lusted after lascivious Lily.

> (P.C. version: Lovely Lulu loved lazy Leonard but he longed for lascivious Lily.)

David danced delightfully and dangerously with a dragon holding a dagger.

Normally there are numerous nerds who are notoriously nutty and nasty.

Tiny Tony tweedled and twirled in his terrific twinkling tutu.

Canadian geese crash gregariously.

Seventy shuddering sailors stood silently as short sharp shattering shocks shook their splendid ship.

Zillions of zebras slithered with suspicion.

The white witch watched the woebegone walrus winding white wool.

Many men.

The monk's monkey mounted the monastery wall and munched melons and macaroni.

Vivacious Vivian vexed ferociously.

Dapper David danced delightfully and dangerously with dainty Dorothy.

Tony tweedled and twirled in his terrific tutu and then took the train to Toronto, then to Timmons, then to Toledo, drinking tequila.

The girl stood on the balustrade balcony, inexplicably mimicking him, hiccuping and amicably welcoming him in.

Red leather, yellow leather.

You need unique New York.

She sells seashells by the seashore.

David danced delightfully and dangerously with Dainty Dorothy, the dragon.

Lovely Lulu loved lazy Leonard.

Tom met Tilly for tea and then took the train to Toledo.

They sang at the singalong until the ding dong rang.

SUMMARY

I have trained over 500 students in the 12 years I have taught at Carnegie Mellon. Some students initially resist the training, as it demands a lot of them in terms of discipline and by asking them to think differently. So teaching this work can be quite challenging, as any voice teacher can attest to. I am, therefore, proud that I frequently receive unsolicited letters and e-mails from students expressing gratitude for the Vox Explora and extolling the value of employing it before auditions and performances. Matthew Bomer (who played the roles of Ben Reade in CBS's *Guiding Light* and Luc in Fox's *Tru Calling*) reported how vital his voice work combined with his yoga practice has been in preparing for television work and helping him stay grounded personally. Dylan Fergus described using the "Vox" regularly while shooting a pilot, and Gaius Charles utilized the Vox Explora in his preparation for his audition for NBC's *Friday Night Lights*, in which he plays the role of Smash Williams.

    On the other hand, I often receive e-mails or calls from students complaining of some vocal problem and seeking my advice. I always ask, "Have you been doing your Vox Explora?" Invariably, the answer is "No." Every time I suggest the same thing, "Remember what I said every class about daily practice? Do your Vox every day for 2 weeks and then contact me again." When they follow this advice, the vocal problem not so magically disappears. Some actors need the experience of vocal trouble before they appreciate the value of the voice work, sometimes causing a certain amount of frustration for the teacher!

    Acting is athletic and the Olympics of voice use. Why would an actor do less than a dancer, or an opera singer, or a musician to prepare? Any director worth his salt will want to reinforce these principles wherever possible.

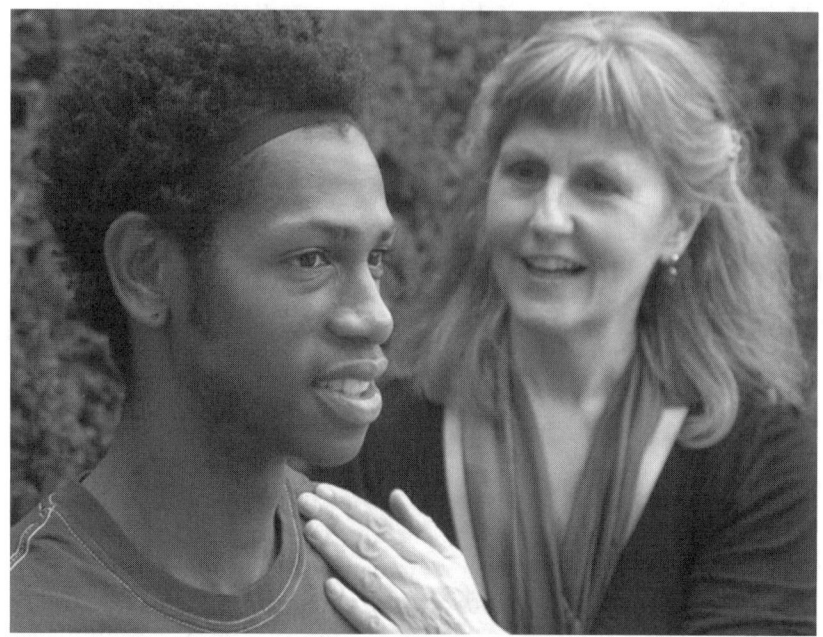
Left to right, Eric Berryman (BFA, Acting student, School of Drama, Carnegie Mellon University) and Janet Madelle Feindel (author). Photo by Karen Waggoner.

CHAPTER 6

Resonex

*R*esonex is a method I developed to give actors specific tools to utilize awareness of resonating areas and then combine this awareness with appropriate text. This provides more vocal choices when one develops a character. Actors learn to differentiate each resonator or resonating area and explore text that highlights the specific characteristics of each resonator. The actor can apply the different resonators to text to investigate less obvious choices within a particular role. Using Resonex increases range and flexibility and the ability to find more emotional nuances in the text, without having to force vocally.

I was first introduced to resonating areas through the work of Kristin Linklater. We explored the six resonators of chest, mouth, teeth, sinus, nasal area, and head on specific sounds, as outlined in her book *Freeing the Natural Voice* (1976). We explored the kinesthetic connection to the sound vibrations in each resonating area and learned to distinguish them. While studying with Linklater in 1993, I was working on a character that I consistently struggled with. I experienced difficulty finding the flow of the character in a manner that I felt at ease with. My characterization felt heavy and self-conscious, in spite of the fact I had actually written the character myself and the other characters seemed to flow well. I had attempted a number of approaches with various coaches and nothing seemed to work. Linklater suggested I do the character allowing my voice to resonate predominantly in the sinus resonator and speak the text faster. To my amazement, the characterization completely changed. I found that the new pace and the sinus resonator allowed for a vocal ease I had never experienced. This created a much more compelling characterization. What I found interesting was the fact that what seemed like an external direction enabled a deeper connection to the text.

When I studied with Robert Palmer at the Royal Academy of Dramatic Art in London, we delved into resonators in a more general way by concentrating on Greek tragedy text excerpts for the chest area, light verse for the mask (resonating area around cheekbones), and then extremely precise text to practice articulation. The teacher emphasized the flexibility needed to tackle the various texts, more than the fact that one used specific resonators. As students, we tended to move into the area instinctively, provided we had vocally warmed up the area sufficiently.

When I began my teaching at Carnegie Mellon, I found the students extremely result-oriented. I taught alongside an excellent teacher who taught from a strict Skinner paradigm that was highly structured. She had a tight curriculum and the students took that work extremely seriously. Prior to my teaching at Carnegie Mellon, I had taught at schools in which the Linklater work was well established, so I had never been in a position where I had to "sell" the importance of the psychophysical work. The Skinner work, at the first-year level, is often presented as rules that need to be rigorously applied to any acting situation with little room for interpretation. First-year undergraduate students often recoil at any sense of ambiguity, so they appreciate the right/wrong methodology. As desperately as these students needed the Linklater work, they simply did not take it seriously. I racked my brains to think of ways to "package" the material so that it would be readily accessible to young undergraduates who had little professional experience and little background in any substantive vocal training. Unfortunately, they did not perceive voice training as a fundamental aspect of the actor's training.

I redesigned my curriculum to make the study of voice more concrete and practical in the hope of motivating my students to dig more deeply into the voice work. I introduced them to the resonating areas based on the Linklater training. Remembering how helpful Robert Palmer's work had been, I examined how one might explore the resonating areas along the Linklater approach and then move on to experiment with texts that lent themselves to the qualities of each specific resonating area. It became evident that certain areas suited different emotional needs within the rhythm, mood, and needs of the text and the character.

My colleague and former teacher, Richard Armstrong, cofounder of the Roy Hart Theatre, describes the voice as a house in which one is constantly discovering new rooms, closets, and cubbyholes. By experimenting with text and resonating areas, the actor becomes more attuned to areas of the voice that she may not use on a regular basis. Experimenting in this way helps the actor strengthen the overall voice as well as the specific areas. It enables the actor to probe into the emotional, psychological, and kinesthetic aspects of the language. Resonex gives actors a way to approach text that in no way interferes with a director's vision.

When I coached at the Stratford Festival in Canada, for example, an actor came to me complaining of hoarseness from the strenuous rehearsals of *Cyrano de Bergerac*. The director had asked him for a "strange" vocal quality. He had approached it the way most actors do when under stress: by tightening in the throat. We experimented and found that he could create the strange quality by employing his nasal resonator while still maintaining his back rib support. This way he was able to give the result the director wanted without causing undue vocal damage. If the text involves an intense high-stakes need, then the chest/back resonating area can help the actor stay grounded and expand to the demands of such a text. If the text involves meticulous and exact use of language, then employing the teeth resonator helps the actor achieve the precision required. Thus, I assign specific texts suited to a particular resonating area for the sound and character qualities that each area tends to embody. This gives the students a tactile feeling of the resonating area as it connects with text, making it more of an acting exercise as well as a voice exercise. The Resonex method serves especially well when the actor needs to make a controversial voice choice. The actor is able to develop specific vocal qualities without vocal strain and to incorporate them into characterizations effectively.

I use Kristin Linklater's resonating areas with a few modifications. One could also apply these to other resonating approaches such as those used in the Roy Hart work. For each area, the student is assigned a piece of text. These can be from different characters from the same play or one can choose different text related to a similar theme. The length should be long enough that the actor can sink her teeth into it but not so long that it becomes difficult to sustain.

Classical texts such as Shakespeare, Restoration, or Greek texts are wonderful to utilize, but one can apply this approach to modern texts with equal success. One group of students used excerpts from *Alice in Wonderland*. Another group used different lines from various sonnets relating to addictive love. In other words, this exercise gives the actor an opportunity to use her creativity.

Remembering that when we refer to voice, what we are really referring to is sound vibrations that move. The actor wants to think of increasing her awareness of particular areas of resonation, rather than becoming too fixed on "placing" the voice. Voice represents sound vibrations that move rather than something that gets fixed in a particular area of resonation. One should think of voice as a verb rather than a noun.

The Resonex method provides a set of tools that one can interchange and rotate as needed.

One needs to understand that one rarely would utilize only one resonator on stage. Generally, actors move through resonators and/or combine resonators. Isolating resonators as an exploration, however, provides an excellent way to examine the landscape and movement of the thoughts.

Choosing the text is an intuitive choice, but here are some of the guidelines for each of the resonators. Please note that Linklater's work generally begins with the chest resonator. I begin with the mouth because many students experience difficulty going directly from the *brumuh-muh-muh* in the Linklater progression into the chest resonator because of the jump to the lower pitch one generally does the chest resonator in. So one can begin in the mouth and then take the pitch down in stages to the chest if necessary.

MOUTH

One uses an open vowel sound on *huh* or [ʌ] in the International Phonetic Alphabet. When employing the mouth resonator, one has a sense of a "round" sound in the middle mouth; the soft palate is lifted fully in what one might refer to as a "plumy" sound. The mouth resonator works well for a high-status character, more formal speech, and/or diplomatic speech. The vowels tend to be long;

the characterization might be slightly pretentious or self-righteous. Ann Bancroft uses considerable mouth resonator in her role as Mrs. Robinson in *The Graduate*. Kristin Scott Thomas uses the mouth resonator to good effect in *Gosford Park* in her role as Sylvia McCord. Albert Hall as Brother Baines in *Malcolm X* is another good example. Following are some text examples.

Twelfth Night, *Orsino's opening speech,*
Act I, Scene i, lines 1–8:

Duke Orsino:
If music be the food of love, play on;
Give me excess of it, that, surfeiting,
The appetite may sicken, and so die.
That strain again! it had a dying fall:
O, it came o'er my ear like the sweet sound,
That breathes upon a bank of violets,
Stealing and giving odour! Enough; no more:
'Tis not so sweet now as it was before.

In this speech, Orsino is slightly in love with himself, the sound of his own voice, and the idea of being in love. The speech is flowery and jumps through different metaphors, mixing up the different senses.

A Midsummer Night's Dream, *Theseus' opening speech*
in Act I, Scene i, lines 1–6, and Hypolyta's response,
lines 7–11:

Theseus:
Now, fair Hippolyta, our nuptial hour
Draws on apace; four happy days bring in
Another moon: but, O, methinks, how slow
This old moon wanes! she lingers my desires,
Like to a step-dame or a dowager
Long withering out a young man's revenue.

Hippolyta:
Four days will quickly steep themselves in night;
Four nights will quickly dream away the time;
And then the moon, like to a silver bow
New-bent in heaven, shall behold the night
Of our solemnities.

The example of Theseus and Hippolyta suits the mouth resonator because they are almost speaking in a coded language. He is saying he wants to make love to her and she is saying, "Just wait a couple of more days, when I am ready." The mouth resonator makes an appropriate diplomatic "cover" with the text.

This is an easier resonator to begin with than the chest/back, because it is easiest to find in the midrange of the voice, which should already be warmed up.

This resonator lends itself to "schmoozing" situations where the character may not actually be expressing the intentions directly or may be embroidering, perhaps a little in love with her own voice. The voice-in-the-mouth resonator might apply to someone a little self-satisfied, like Gary Essendine in *Present Laughter* by Noel Coward, Act I:

> Listen to me, my dearest. You're not in love with me—the real me. You're in love with an illusion, the illusion that I gave you when you saw me on the stage. Last night I ran the risk of breaking that dear young illusion forever—but I didn't—it's still there. I can see it in your eyes but never again—never never again—moments like last night—that's all I dare hope for now—that's why I'm so lonely, so desperately lonely, but I have learned one bitter lesson in my life and that lesson is to be able to say goodbye.

Here the character has a melodramatic and smarmy quality that the actor can play with, using the mouth resonator. It is extremely important that, even while the actor is exploring awareness of sound vibrations in a particular area, she keeps strongly connected to the meaning and intention through the specific use of the language.

CHEST/BACK RESONATOR: PRAYING TO THE GODS AND GODDESSES

For this resonator, one uses an open vowel sound—*hah* or [ha] in phonetics. Generally, this is meant to be at the lower end in the pitch of one's range. One can bring the pitch down gradually, starting at middle-C range in women and low-C range in men, to help ease into the lower pitch range without pushing. The trick is to keep thinking of the release of the sound emitting from the whole body and remembering that the spine lengthens on the release of sound. It also helps to imagine the sound moving out from the sternum in front of the body and out between the shoulder blades in the back. One can imagine the sound coming up from the feet and spiraling around the body through the front and back. This image helps actors eschew the tendency to pull down and squeeze on the release of sound. Some actors are under the faulty notion this pulling down and squeezing increases intensity when, in fact, it only causes constriction in the laryngeal area, which can eventually cause vocal damage.

To explore the chest/back resonator, the actor drops the head back from the occipital area. One can imagine one is moving one's head up and over a greasy pole that goes through one's ears, keeping the back of the neck long. This allows the neck to remain free so as not to constrict in the larynx area. Then one lifts the arms over the head in a *V* shape, moving the arms slightly forward, thinking of the back muscles connecting to the arms, with energy out the fingers. The arms should not be held stiffly nor should they be too lax. The actor imagines asking "the gods" for something on "hah" so that the sound is motivated. Asking the gods for something also encourages largess without pushing. It reminds us of our relationship to the cosmos, particularly valuable in classical plays.

Text suitable for this resonator tends toward the more vocally challenging, that is, moments in plays where the intensity is high and actors want to go into "pushing mode" or "play for the emotion rather than the intention mode." A text that requires a great deal of grounding and strength is most suitable to use to strengthen this area. The actor must be very conscious of supporting the specifics of text and using expansiveness in the back intercostal muscles and rib area. Suitable text tends to be high stakes moments, when a character really has to speak her truth for the first time. Or the character may need to defend herself or her honor. Generally, these moments involve a direct line between the actor's guts and the actor's words—no embroidery, no masking or hiding behind the words but using the words to pursue truth in a high stakes situation. Often, this resonator is useful when speaking to the gods, the cosmos, or the heavens. A good example of this is Denzel Washington in *Malcolm X*, part II, when he is addressing the crowd in Harlem and says, " . . . as what I am—a Black man." He drops fully into his chest resonator, giving enormous weight to what he says. Through this speech, he moves through all his resonators, but in certain sections really takes advantage of his rich chest resonance, which gives him great authority, when he needs it in this scene.

Here are some examples of Shakespearean texts suited to the chest/back resonator.

Twelfth Night, *Act V, Scene i, lines 66-86, Antonio's speech to Sebastian*:

Antonio:
Orsino, noble sir,
Be pleased that I shake off these names you give me:
Antonio never yet was thief or pirate,
Though I confess, on base and ground enough,
Orsino's enemy. A witchcraft drew me hither:
That most ingrateful boy there by your side,
From the rude sea's enraged and foamy mouth
Did I redeem; a wrack past hope he was:
His life I gave him and did thereto add
My love, without retention or restraint,
All his in dedication; for his sake
Did I expose myself, pure for his love,
Into the danger of this adverse town;
Drew to defend him when he was beset:
Where being apprehended, his false cunning,
Not meaning to partake with me in danger,
Taught him to face me out of his acquaintance,
And grew a twenty years removed thing
While one would wink; denied me mine own purse,
Which I had recommended to his use
Not half an hour before.

A Midsummer Night's Dream, *Oberon and Titania, Act II, Scene i, lines 60-81*:

Oberon:
Ill met by moonlight, proud Titania.

Titania:
What, jealous Oberon! Fairies, skip hence:
I have forsworn his bed and company.

Oberon:
Tarry, rash wanton: am not I thy lord?

Titania:
Then I must be thy lady: but I know
When thou hast stolen away from fairy land,
And in the shape of Corin sat all day,
Playing on pipes of corn and versing love
To amorous Phillida. Why art thou here,
Come from the farthest Steppe of India?
But that, forsooth, the bouncing Amazon,
Your buskin'd mistress and your warrior love,
To Theseus must be wedded, and you come
To give their bed joy and prosperity.

Oberon:
How canst thou thus for shame, Titania,
Glance at my credit with Hippolyta,
Knowing I know thy love to Theseus?
Didst thou not lead him through the glimmering night
From Perigenia, whom he ravished?
And make him with fair Aegles break his faith,
With Ariadne and Antiopa?

Titania:
These are the forgeries of jealousy . . .

King Lear, *Act III, Scene ii, lines 1-9*:

King Lear:
Blow, winds, and crack your cheeks! rage! blow!
You cataracts and hurricanoes, spout
Till you have drench'd our steeples, drown'd the cocks!
You sulphurous and thought-executing fires,
Vaunt-couriers to oak-cleaving thunderbolts,
Singe my white head! And thou, all-shaking thunder,
Smite flat the thick rotundity o' the world!
Crack nature's moulds, all germens spill at once,
That make ingrateful man!

Lear is communicating with Nature and needs to release the thoughts to a force much greater than him.

Here one should choose texts to do with a character asserting herself; making a claim; speaking a truism that may be frustrating and/or painful; or a situation in which the character erupts. When teaching this resonator, one may use the image of "keening"— expressing grieving, as if one is moaning on the *hah*. We refer to this as "praying to the gods or goddesses or God," whatever the individual chooses. If one is doing it as part of a group, it can be fun for the group to "affirm" something together such as a good performance, support for someone in trouble, and so on. This is a good way to get into a lower pitched scream as well. One can start with the *hah* and then increase the need for expression to sustain it into a moan, and then into a scream, allowing the sound to resonate freely through the whole body. It is extremely important to keep the back open here by thinking of the sound releasing out the back, keeping length through the body.

TEETH

The actor goes back to the mouth resonator—which will make the transition into the teeth resonator easier—and then to the teeth resonating area.

With the teeth resonator, the head drops slightly forward, the sound releasing on the open vowel of *hee* or [hi]. Here the difficulty is that the actor may tend to push the sound by tightening in the tongue root. The actor can think of a conveyor belt of sound, with the sound impulse starting at the back ribs, moving along the back and up along the hard palate, through the teeth. The actor then returns to the mouth resonator, as a neutral place.

This resonator lends itself to texts that require extreme precision. This is a fun resonator for exploring Restoration text, quickly paced verse, or a text that conveys orders. If a passage uses many consonants, then this resonator is particularly helpful.

Jeremy Northam in his role as Sir Robert Morton in *The Winslow Boy* provides an excellent example of the use of the teeth resonator in the scene in which he meets the accused boy for the first time and aggressively interrogates him. Once he has decided the boy is innocent, he seamlessly switches back to the mouth resonator, perfectly maintaining his undeniable high status in the scene. Other Shakespearean examples include the following.

Twelfth Night, *Act III, Scene ii, lines 60-65*:

Maria:
If you desire the spleen, and will laugh yourself
into stitches, follow me. Yond gull Malvolio is

turned heathen, a *very* renegado; for there is no
Christian, that means to be saved by believing
rightly, can ever believe such impossible passages
of grossness. He's in yellow stockings.

This resonator gives a sense of urgency and distinctness; it is useful for conspiratorial speeches, such as Angelo's in *Measure for Measure*, Act II, Scene iv, lines 154-170:

Angelo:
Who will believe thee, Isabel?
My unsoil'd name, the austereness of my life,
My vouch against you, and my place i' the state,
Will so your accusation overweigh,
That you shall stifle in your own report
And smell of calumny. I have begun,
And now I give my sensual race the rein:
Fit thy consent to my sharp appetite;
Lay by all nicety and prolixious blushes,
That banish what they sue for; redeem thy brother
By yielding up thy body to my will;
Or else he must not only die the death,
But thy unkindness shall his death draw out
To lingering sufferance. Answer me to-morrow,
Or, by the affection that now guides me most,
I'll prove a tyrant to him. As for you,
Say what you can, my false o'erweighs your true.

Here the teeth resonator helps convey the threatening quality of Angelo in the scene with Isabel. He uses the words like venom, spitting his vile thoughts at her.

Y<small>BUZZ</small>

After exploring the teeth resonator with precision of thought and the text, the actor then moves to the *Ybuzz*, the Arthur Lessac exercise (although here we may be using a slightly higher pitch— slightly higher than the pitch of one's habitual speaking voice—than he uses). The actor imagines the sound moving along the conveyor belt again, but this time the actor should feel the resonance in the alveolar ridge (or gum ridge) and the area above the upper lip (moustache). This resonator is especially helpful for British or French accents, mask work, and those for whom articulation is difficult.

The vowel sound is the diphthong *yee-ee-ee* or [yi: i: i:]. It is very close to the teeth, but gives a slightly sexier quality because one is engaging the lips in a bit of a pout. One thinks of the sound emitting through the alveolar ridge through the upper lip area. I often use an image for this resonator of a Folies Bergère dancer or the naughty French maid. There is a rather mischievous quality to this sound, as if one is onto something, a sense of discovery. In HBO's *The Sopranos*, Tony Soprano's Russian girlfriend, Irina, played by actress Oksana Lada, utilizes this resonator a great deal, particularly in the scene where he insists she see a psychiatrist and she responds with, "You're not the boss of me" (Green, Burgess, & Coulter, 2000). In *Sex and the City* (Kohan & Seidelman, 1998), Carrie Bradshaw meets a Euro-trash call girl, Amalita Amalfi, played by Carole Davis, and jet-setting French architect Gilles (played by Ed Fry), who both tell Carrie (played by Sarah Jessica Parker) that she "eez dee most beauteeful woman in New York" in a perfect Ybuzz resonator. This resonator is particularly useful in preparation for certain dialects and accents, such as British or French, in which the sound placement is more forward than General American. Following are some text examples, which are played in General American, but the Ybuzz can add a fun component to the exploration of the Shakespeare text. Titania here no longer holds the great authority she does in her first scene with Oberon. After Oberon casts the love spell on her and she wakes up to find Bottom and falls in love with him, she becomes positively silly as she dotes on him.

A Midsummer Night's Dream, *Act III, Scene 1, lines 124-128*:

Titania:
I pray thee, gentle mortal, sing again:
Mine ear is much enamour'd of thy note;
So is mine eye enthralled to thy shape;
And thy fair virtue's force perforce doth move me
On the first view to say, to swear, I love thee.

Twelfth Night, *Malvolio, Act III, Scene iv, lines 18-21*:

Malvolio:
Sad, lady? I could be sad: this does make some obstruction in the blood, this cross-gartering; but what of that? If it please the

eye of one, it is with me as the very true sonnet is, "Please one, and please all."

Malvolio here becomes embarrassingly brazen with Olivia, and the Ybuzz helps the actor to find the freedom to do this.

Sinus

The actor moves on to the sinus area, just below the cheekbones. The soft palate is raised. This area allows for vulnerability. One must explore this extremely gently on the sound *hee* or [hi].

This sound/area has a fragile, unaffected quality and is especially useful in the exploration of text dealing with discovery, magic, and/or love. Mia Farrow uses this resonator a lot in her portrayal of Rosemary in *Rosemary's Baby*. Other examples follow.

In this first example, from Shakespeare's *King Lear*, Cordelia speaks the truth from her heart. The delivery is simple and vulnerable.

King Lear, *Cordelia, Act I, Scene i, lines 91-104*:

Cordelia:
Unhappy that I am, I cannot heave
My heart into my mouth: I love your majesty
According to my bond; nor more nor less . . .
(Lear speaks)
Good my lord,
You have begot me, bred me, loved me: I
Return those duties back as are right fit,
Obey you, love you, and most honour you.
Why have my sisters husbands, if they say
They love you all? Haply, when I shall wed,
That lord whose hand must take my plight shall carry
Half my love with him, half my care and duty:
Sure, I shall never marry like my sisters,
To love my father all.

In the following example, it is a wonderful turning point in the play when Sebastian and Viola recognize each other. There is a metaphysical quality that the sinus resonator lends itself to: the possibility that the one Viola thought was dead is really alive and that she is not who she seems to be.

Twelfth Night, *Sebastian and Viola:* Act V, Scene i, lines 219-250:

Sebastian:
Do I stand there? I never had a brother;
Nor can there be that deity in my nature,
Of here and every where. I had a sister,
Whom the blind waves and surges have devour'd.
Of charity, what kin are you to me?
What countryman? what name? what parentage?

Viola:
Of Messaline: Sebastian was my father;
Such a Sebastian was my brother too,
So went he suited to his watery tomb:
If spirits can assume both form and suit
You come to fright us.

Sebastian:
A spirit I am indeed;
But am in that dimension grossly clad
Which from the womb I did participate.
Were you a woman, as the rest goes even,
I should my tears let fall upon your cheek,
And say "Thrice-welcome, drowned Viola!"

Viola:
My father had a mole upon his brow.

Sebastian:
And so had mine.

Viola:
And died that day when Viola from her birth
Had number'd thirteen years.

Sebastian:
O, that record is lively in my soul!
He finished indeed his mortal act
That day that made my sister thirteen years.

Viola:
If nothing lets to make us happy both
But this my masculine usurp'd attire,
Do not embrace me till each circumstance
Of place, time, fortune, do cohere and jump
That I am Viola: which to confirm,

I'll bring you to a captain in this town,
Where lie my maiden weeds; by whose gentle help
I was preserved to serve this noble count.
All the occurrence of my fortune since
Hath been between this lady and this lord.

In the following scene, the Princess has just heard of her father's death, which jolts her into a more sober adulthood and responsibility. She speaks these lines with care but with honesty. The sinus resonator expresses the lines with simplicity, without any masking. (Of course one could make the choice to make the Princess more covered in her delivery, and use a bit of the mouth resonator as a cover to the shock of her father's death—or a combination of both.)

Love's Labor's Lost, *Act V, Scene ii, lines 767-774*:

Princess:
We have received your letters full of love;
Your favours, the ambassadors of love;
And, in our maiden council, rated them
At courtship, pleasant jest and courtesy,
As bombast and as lining to the time:
But more devout than this in our respects
Have we not been; and therefore met your loves
In their own fashion, like a merriment.

There is a fragile quality to this resonating area. It is useful for exploring a moment in which the character exposes herself.

NASAL

The nasal area involves the sound resonating in the bridge of the nose. One must approach this resonator extra gently, as it is easy to strain here.

Additionally, one must be careful not to push this too vigorously, as it can result in tightening at the tongue root and resulting tension in the throat. Rather than go right into the pingy *mee-mee-mee-mee-mee, may-may-may-may-may, mi-mi-mi-mi-mi (long vowel here)* I suggest using a gentler humming version first: *mee, may, mah, mo, moo* [mi-mai-ma-mo-mu:]. The next step is massaging the tongue root, adding a stronger resonance at the bridge of the nose. One can always think of a yawn to keep the throat open.

This resonator is called the *elf* or the *violin* in the Roy Hart work. The actor uses the image of the character of the elf to get in touch with the emotional qualities of this resonator. The actor can also chant the word *violin*, sensing the sound pinging on the bridge of the nose. The nasal resonator carries extremely well. It fills a large space, right to the back of a theater. One must balance it with the other resonators in order for the sound quality not to become too overwhelming for an audience. When this resonator dominates, it can become rather irritating; that said, however, it adds a lovely ironic flavor to characterizations. It is a fun resonator to add flavor for clown or comic purposes. Some of the world's most respected actors employ a fair bit of nasal resonance to excellent ironic effect: Maggie Smith as Constance Trentham in her line in *Gosford Park*, "tricky color green—very tricky"; Jack Nicholson as Garrett Breedlove in *Terms of Endearment* when he says to Shirley MacLaine's character, Aurora Greenway, "Almost made a clean getaway"; and James Gandolfini as Tony Soprano, to name but a few. As one is exploring the sound, one can think of whining or a dog moaning before a thunderstorm on a gentle hum. Some Shakespeare text examples follow.

King Lear, *Act III, Scene ii, lines 25-36*:

The Fool:
He that has a house to put 's head in has a good
head-piece.
    The cod-piece that will house
    Before the head has any,
    The head and he shall louse;
    So beggars marry many.
    The man that makes his toe
    What he his heart should make
    Shall of a corn cry woe,
    And turn his sleep to wake.
For there was never yet fair woman but she made
mouths in a glass.

A Midsummer Night's Dream, *Act III, Scene i, lines 129–133*:

Bottom:
Methinks, mistress, you should have little reason
for that: and yet, to say the truth, reason and

love keep little company together now-a-days; the more the pity that some honest neighbors will not make them friends. Nay, I can gleek upon occasion.

This example of Bottom is especially successful because it involves a lot of nasal sounds, which add a rather "neighing" quality.

It can be used in more serious pieces to add nasal quality to evoke an irony as mentioned above. It would be useful for Iago in *Othello* or the title role in *Richard III* (think of Laurence Olivier in this role, in which he combined the nasal and teeth to good effect).

SNASAL

This is a resonator that came out of class exploration by combining nasal and sinus. A fabulous example of the *snasal* resonator is in *The Sopranos'* second season, episode 24 (Winter & Van Patten, 2002) in a scene where Junior has caught his hand in the drain in the kitchen sink and Janice (actress Aida Turturro) and Richie (actor David Proval) come in to find him. As Richie helps Junior get his hand out of the sink, he says, "Relax, you're flexing, you're flexing." Joe Pesci has often used this resonator, particularly in the movie *Casino*.

This resonator is especially useful for "tough guy" characters. As with the nasal and head, the support is paramount because the tendency is to push for the sound. The way to prevent this is to imagine the sound out the back of the head, a trick I learned when I coached at the Stratford Festival in Canada from the talented actress Barbara Bryne, whose voice could always be heard with clarity and complete ease in the 1,800-seat thrust theater.

HEAD

In the Linklater work, one employs the sound *kee* to explore the head resonator. One imagines the sound emitting from around the skull, as if one's head was made of gauze, or one was wearing a cap used for streaking one's hair. It is important that the sound remain extremely gentle. Using this resonator helps remind actors to lift the soft palate. It is extremely important to maintain proper breath support well in all these resonator explorations. It may even be helpful to expand the intercostal muscles, provided one keeps the shoulders and neck muscles released. This is due to the fact that this resonator is high in pitch—about high C for women and low C for men on the piano scale. For men, one can use falsetto, or, as Richard Armstrong would say, "true" setto.

Linklater teaches that strengthening this resonator strengthens the lower pitch range as well as the higher pitches and increases flexibility in all the resonator work. The head selections need to be short in length, as, because of its intensity, this resonator can be difficult to sustain.

Useful for the head resonator are exclamatory and urgent texts. It is rare that in actual performance an actor would use exclusively this resonator. Mira Sorvino uses a clever combination of head and nasal in her role as Linda in *Mighty Aphrodite*. At the end of the movie, in the final scene with Woody Allen, she alters her voice, making it sound more grounded, less nasal and less head, and lower in pitch, which accurately reflects the evolution of her character. Another example in Shakespeare well suited to this resonator follows.

Twelfth Night, *Sir Andrew, Act V, Scene i, lines 166-171*:

Sir Andrew:
For the love of God, a surgeon! Send one presently to Sir Toby.

[Olivia:
What's the matter?]

Sir Andrew:
He has broke my head across and has given Sir Toby a bloody coxcomb too. For the love of God, your help.

Othello, *Act V, Scene ii, lines 123-125*:

Emilia:
Out, and alas! that was my lady's voice.
Help! help, ho! help! O lady, speak again!
Sweet Desdemona! O sweet mistress, speak!

With this resonator, the actor must support and release the sound, imagining the sound starting at the feet and then coming out of the skull, keeping the shoulder and neck muscles as released as possible. It is important to keep the intention extremely specific, crying for help or whatever it is, and not just go for a generic sound.

Breaking the resonators down in this manner allows detailed, specific exploration and gives the actor more options, but I must emphasize that these are tools along the way. One would not limit oneself to one resonator under normal circumstances, but having broken the resonators down allows actors to develop more vocal options by strengthening individual areas. Then the actor can let go and simply allow the voice to respond to the needs and thoughts of the characters spontaneously with the underpinnings of the range of possibilities.

Tools for Rehearsals

In a rehearsal process, a director might utilize Resonex in the following ways:

- Go through a particular text from a specific play, encouraging the actors to impose a resonator that they might not necessarily employ habitually. Sometimes it can be interesting to go against what one expects (that is, pick a resonator that would not be the most obvious choice) to see what new discoveries might occur. The next step is to repeat the scenes without imposing the resonator consciously, to see what one can discover in terms of wider range, flexibility, and vocal freedom.

- Go through one monologue or scene and as an *exploration*, work through specific resonating areas, as the thoughts change in the piece. This can provide a useful approach to text analysis. For example, in the opening monologue in *Richard III*, one might start in mouth, as he speaks rather diplomatically lines 1 to 8. As Richard speaks lines 9 to 12 ("grim visaged war . . . ") one might move into teeth, spitting the thoughts out as Richard works himself up into the lines "to the lascivious pleasing of a lute. . . . " The next thoughts from lines 13 to 17 ("But, I, that am not shaped for sportive tricks, nor made to court an amorous looking glass . . . ") could be nasal, going into head on line 18 ("I, that am curtailed of this fair proportion . . . ") to line 23 ("That dogs bark at me as I halt by them") and so on.

The important thing is to use the resonator as a tool for meaning and mood. After encouraging the actor to explore the text in this way several times, ask the actor to perform it in a "free-flow" fashion; that is, not imposing anything on it and seeing how the prior exploration informs the text and playing.

Another option is for actors to play scenes, changing resonators each time the actor changes a tactic. Or the actors can employ a new resonator each time the status changes between characters. Similarly, one can employ a new resonator each time a new piece of information is introduced. The goal is to become more flexible and allow more possibilities in terms of character and emotion and allow the voice to reflect those changes. Again, one then wants to run the scene or scenes without imposing the resonator changes, but just allowing the actors to respond spontaneously. In general, one finds that the actors then discover more depth in their connection to the text as well as more variety and freedom vocally. In rehearsal, this helps actors and directors to "get out of the box" in their thinking as well as bring a sense of play to the proceedings.

Here are some ways teachers can integrate Resonex into classroom or studio explorations with text:

- Students explore specific areas of resonance on open sound, and then work on individually, out loud, experimenting with using particular resonators on specific points in the text, as fitting to the intentions and meaning. They can then develop a Resonex color-coded text and work on really exaggerating each resonating area, while maintaining their support and a strong intention within that structure. Then they take the text again (free-flow version) and see how the Resonex version informs their delivery. Generally, they find a much more organic connection to the language in their free-flow version, and hence more vocal freedom and flexibility by using parts of their range they don't normally engage. This is particularly helpful when someone tends toward a monotone delivery.

- Students are assigned a play and then must choose monologues that best represent the characteristics of each resonator. This forces them to grapple with the meaning of the play and make decisions about how that meaning is best conveyed. Often, there may be a number of choices, so this can stimulate lively discussions as well.

- Combine writing and Resonex: Actors write a few lines or monologues using particular resonators, developing particular characters for each area. This can also be useful for voice-over and animation copy as "a way in." They pick a theme and have different Resonex character voices within an overall context. For example, one student did the Emmy Awards, with a variety of acceptance speeches, each one utilizing a specific area. As mentioned earlier, students have developed pieces with great imagination. They get so involved with the story and the characters that they learn to master the technical challenges in an individual and creative way. As one explores these, one develops new ways to mix up exercises in original ways.

A former student, the gifted Demetrius Gross, wrote a brilliant piece about eight men already on death row and accused of murdering someone in the prison. He used the mouth resonator for an eloquent Black Muslim character, the Ybuzz resonator for a campy character, chest/back for the bullying guard, nasal for a drugged-out character, and so on. It was moving, funny, and deeply disturbing. Gross embodied each character beautifully. He continued to develop it during his time at Carnegie Mellon, and I would ask him to perform it annually for the first-year acting students. He delved more and more deeply into the characterizations, and the piece became more and more powerful. He really could develop it into a complete show. It certainly held the bar high for the first-year students.

Another student, Kersti Bryan, played a tooth community, with Pearl White as a front tooth, a Grace Kelly-type character; a hard hitting Texan as a lower molar; the teeth resonator as a cultivated East Indian running for mayor, promising to get rid of gingivitis; and the head resonator as a rotting tooth in the back of the mouth. The theme centered on which tooth personality was responsible for the gingivitis. It was hilarious. Bryan is now acting with the company of the Oregon Shakespeare Festival, but I can't help but wonder if she might write imaginative commercials some day.

The structure of the Resonex stimulated wonderful creativity in the students. When I first introduced this to the first-year voice class at Carnegie Mellon in 1999, Joshua Gad (a 2003 grad who recently played the lead in *Spelling Bee* on Broadway and other roles including Bump in *Mardi Gras* (director Phil Dornfeld, writer Josh Herald, produced by Columbia Pictures) wrote an Original Resonex involving a number of movie stars: Jack Nicholson as the nasal character, and an impression in the chest/back of my colleague, actor/director/writer/teacher Tony McKay, associate professor and former head of acting, School of Drama, Carnegie Mellon University.

Matthew Griffin (with roles including ones on HBO's *Entourage* and *Cashmere Mafia* and CBS's *NUMB3RS*) and Leslie Odom, Jr. (recurring roles on ABC's *Big Day* (Fred) and *CSI Miami*) led an improvisation in class in which they switched around all eight resonators as they depicted a family at dinner, stuffing themselves with too much food.

Laura Mixon, another student, wrote a piece that took place in a flower bed, where the flowers were competing over who would be the representative at the social gathering in honor of the Higher Power. The snasal character was the garlic, shunned by all; the pansy was the sinus, extremely vulnerable and experiencing awful discrimination from some of the other characters for being gay; and the rose character was played in the mouth resonator as a kind of upper-crust socialite snob with a sense of entitlement. It was a hilarious, profound, and imaginative piece of social commentary.

Another student, Kyle Beltran, wrote a piece in which each resonator defined a character in a hospital waiting room dealing with life-and-death issues. It was both funny and poignant. Another student, Bernie Balbot, played a variety of types of candies. Gabriel King created a film noir mystery piece in which the main detective was played in the chest resonator, the female heroine in the Ybuzz, and so on.

The writing really helps the actors connect with their imagination and the need to communicate. The actors find more ease and vocal freedom when they combine the writing with the exploration of the resonators because they become so focused on what they are saying and less self-conscious about the voice. They also develop useful tools to take into a rehearsal process, particularly when playing a number of characters within a play. In guiding actors with this work, it's important for them to go fully into each character and not make them caricatures. Thus, it helps the actor build a strong foundation, combining sound with thought.

SUMMARY

By employing and adapting the principles of Resonex in a rehearsal, directors can open up possibilities in text and emotional freedom within the text. The Resonex approach is particularly helpful during the early period of rehearsal, especially if a scene or an actor seems stuck. Resonex allows actors to examine different aspects of the scene in a way that is creative, encouraging spontaneity and freedom. The Resonex is also a useful tool for text analysis, and encourages vocal flexibility without self-consciousness. Once the actor explores the text with the Resonex and then takes the text without imposing that, the actor finds more freedom and ease.

One might compare the voice to a big house with lots of rooms, and exploring the resonators helps actors discover some rooms they are not familiar with and increase awareness of those they know well. The Resonex is easily adapted for modern, classical, and physically based acting, and develops the psychophysical connection to voice by freeing up the imagination and the actor's inner resources.

CHAPTER 7

Voice and Text Explorations

In order to guide actors in integrating the principles of healthy voice usage, the director should develop and maintain a vocabulary and methodology. The director should also reinforce the work of the voice and text coach wherever possible.

There are many excellent texts available with which directors should familiarize themselves, most notably *From Word to Play* (2008), *Text in Action* (2001), and *The Actor and the Text* (2000) by Cicely Berry, O.B.E., Director of Voice at the Royal Shakespeare Company in England. In all three books, Berry details excellent ways to help the actor develop a more visceral connection to language and thought.

One basic principle is that the director needs to emphasize the importance of playing intention, as opposed to giving suggestions that emphasize "state of being" notes such as "The character is angry." The director should reinforce the idea of "the thought propelling the sound" and, in general, avoid notes such as "This is how to say this" or "This is the word to hit." If the actor becomes too focused on the external and result-oriented note, the actor will lose the organic rhythm of the language, which comes from a response to the actor's intention. Directors therefore must be careful to reinforce this delicate balance and think carefully about the notes they give. When a director gives an emotional note, the actor almost always pushes vocally in order to achieve the desired result, and then the result does not read believably. *A Practical Handbook for the Actor* (Bruder et al., 1986) has some good suggestions for making notes actable. Of particular interest is the chapter entitled "The Emotional Trap," which offers useful suggestions on how to avoid the pitfall of playing an emotion and ways to "reframe" emotional notes to help the actor find more action-oriented ways of interpreting directors' suggestions. Directors can learn from this chapter and frame notes in a manner that is more helpful to actors and to actors' voices. I remember studying with Cicely Berry when she told the group, "Emotion is boring. It's much more interesting to watch the movement of the thought."[1]

In her book *The Actor and the Text* (2000), Cicely Berry refers to the delicate balance inherent in the energy of the language. The actor does not need to push, muscle, and/or squeeze the text for meaning nor approach it so casually that the natural vitality of the text is flattened.

> But whatever the style of the writing, the actor has to find the right energy for that particular text; if his energy becomes too inward and controlled the words become dull; if he presses too much energy out the words will be unfocused and the thought will be generalized. (p. 9)
>
> Ideally, I suppose, every actor wants to know that his voice is carrying what is in his mind and imagination directly across to the audience. He wants it to be accurate in his intention and to sound unforced. (p. 14)

In her book (2000), Berry outlines many exercises designed to help the actor connect to the kinesthetic energy within the language. Through these various physical explorations with text, the actor taps into a more intuitive relationship to the language and the dynamic movement of thought with the voice resounding from a deeper place in both the body and psyche.

It is easy, as an actor, to get caught up in the emotion and think to oneself, "Oh, I am really feeling this, so it must be good." This, however, misleads the actor, as it distracts us from the task at hand, which is pursuing the intention and moving the action and thoughts forward in the play.

---

[1] Voice and Speech Trainers Voice/Text workshop led by Cicely Berry and Andrew Wade, organized by Barbara Acker, PhD, Phoenix, Arizona, January 1994.

Here is an example I experienced while participating in the above-mentioned workshop led by Cicely Berry and Andrew Wade. I was working on scene 10 in *A Streetcar Named Desire* by Tennessee Williams. This is the scene in which Stanley returns home after Stella has given birth, and Blanche is alone with Stanley in the apartment. Berry put a number of items on the table and told me I had to protect them and not to let the actor playing Stanley take any of them away from me. We did the scene, and he attempted to take these things away. I grabbed them and clung to them as tightly as I was able. The words began to have a much stronger resonance and I tapped into Blanche's tremendous strength, which previously I had not been aware of. The objects I was protecting represented my independence and dignity that Stanley was doing his best to bully out of me. Often, one approaches such a part by focusing on the instability of the character, trying to "show" the fragile emotional state of Blanche to the audience instead of putting the attention on the desperate will of the character to overcome her circumstances and mental state in order to succeed and normalize her situation. This, of course, makes the conflict much more interesting. Blanche is not trying to show how "crazy" she is, but trying to find balance and a safe haven in her life, and Stanley represents the obstacle to this.

While studying with Berry and Wade, I witnessed a woman deliver a monologue of Lady Macbeth's. One might describe the performance attempt as histrionic. It was extremely tight, overemotional, and difficult to listen to. Berry asked the actress to pick up all the shoes of the participants in the workshop in the room, sequentially. As she spoke her text, the actress walked around the room, picking up the shoes and putting them into a pile. The actress's vocal delivery suddenly became animated, charming, and totally engaging; all while she was organizing the shoes. Her voice resonated with ease and full support, and the previous tension was gone.

What happened? Berry calls these *diversion tactics*. The task of putting the shoes in order took the actress's attention off the end result, thus preventing her habitual response to the delivery of text and allowing her to discover the inherent freedom within the energy of the text itself. One might say she got out of the way of the text, letting the text play her. Instead of imposing her own preconceived idea of the way the text should play and manipulating her delivery, she found a more intuitive connection to the language. By taking the attention off the result, ironically, the outcome proved far more interesting to the listener.

There exist many similar exercises to "take the weight off the text."

Here's a similar example. In a rehearsal of *Love's Labor's Lost*, directed by Robin Phillips at the Stratford Festival in Canada,[2] I observed the following exercise designed to address this issue. In Act 5, scene 2, Phillips asked the actresses to play the scene as if they were pinning their hair up with bobby pins. When the actresses put imaginary bobby pins in their hair, the scene played lighter and funnier. The voices became freer and more expressive. Putting attention on the bobby pins took some unneeded weight off the text, allowing the delivery of the lines to be more natural. When the actresses went back to play the scene again, this time without miming pinning their hair up, they were able to maintain the same lightness and freedom. Because these were such talented actors (Martha Henry, Domini Blythe, Barbara March, and Barbara Stuart), their own instincts incorporated the kinesthetic memory of what they had discovered. They were then able to integrate the new information into the scene successfully.

The members of Shakespeare & Company[3] have developed and refined an exercise called "dropping in" to explore and help free the subconscious energy of the language. The coach (or director) and actor work together as the actor repeats specific words in the text while the coach asks questions and comments. If the word were *winter* in the line, "Now is the winter of our discontent," from *Richard III*, the coach might feed suggestions by asking questions like, "What does your skin feel like when it's cold?" "Do you feel isolated in winter?" "Does the wind bite through you during the winter?" "What is absent in winter?" and so on. The actor continues to repeat the word *winter*, each time gaining a deeper emotional connection to the word as he experiences the impact of each question. Another example might be the word *mother*. The coach might ask questions such as, "How close are you to your mother?" "Do you miss your mother?" or simply feed the actor images: "breast," "feed," "comfort," "criticism," "love," and so on. The coach and actor go through each word in this way, with the exception of words such as *in* and *that*. Then the actor goes back and repeats the full line of

---

[2]Stratford Shakespeare Festival, Stratford, Ontario, Canada, 1979.
[3]Founded by Tina Packer, Dennis Krausnick, and Kristin Linklater, Lenox, Massachusetts, in 1967.

text, having dropped in each word. The actor generally connects to the meaning of the text more fully because of a deeper kinesthetic and emotional relationship to the words.

At Shakespeare & Company, the company members drop in the text of a whole production. It can be equally effective to drop in a section of text (of about 10-15 lines) thoroughly. The discoveries unearthed from doing that smaller section will still bleed into other sections of the play. Though not quite as effective, actors can also explore the text on their own, repeating each word with eyes closed and free-associating as they say each word. One must remember, however, that this is not a substitute for the more analytical text work one must do in preparation for rehearsal and performance.

The following section includes examples of ways to explore text to help the actor gain a more visceral connection to the language and intention of a particular character. The voice and text work by Cicely Berry, Kristin Linklater, Andrew Wade, Francis Thomas, Tina Packer, Dennis Krausnick, David Smukler, and Patsy Rodenburg inspire many of these, and I have synthesized these ideas with my own approach.

The best way to approach these exercises is in the spirit of experimentation—"Let's see what we find," rather than grasping too hard for specific results. Each exercise should be explored fully, and then the actor should go back to the text, without imposing but allowing the experience of the exploration to inform the delivery. One should not hang onto the discovery, but allow the new information to cook in the actor's subconscious, and hopefully the actor will integrate what is helpful for the performance.

Text Explorations

If the actor is rushing through the text and having trouble really giving the images their full weight:

- Have the actor say the text with eyes closed, and visualize each image fully before speaking it. Then have him speak the same text with eyes open. Generally, this heightens the awareness of the visual imagery. It is important to encourage the actor to really see the image and not speak until the image becomes specific. The tone of the voice and the support often change dramatically.

- Have the actor make a collage of the text, being careful to illustrate each specific image. This helps the actor to become intimately connected with each image and is particularly useful with Shakespeare, particularly for those who have not acted Shakespeare a great deal before. (This exercise is particularly useful in a training situation.)

- Have the actor draw each event and image, like an animation cartoon, as the actor is speaking the text. Often the actor discovers he has been glossing over parts of the text. Then have the actor repeat the text again and look for the new discoveries.

- Have the actor mime each image of the text and then speak the text after exploring it in this way.

- Have the actor actually draw something else as she speaks the text and then speak the text again, without the activity, and see how this informs the delivery.

If the actor is tending to be too "small" in his interpretation:

- Suggest he mime painting each image on a huge canvas with large movements, making sure to include the back awareness. Then the actor delivers the text again, without the movements. This generally helps the actor find the expansiveness of the images and incorporate them into the performance.

- Ask the actor to play the monologue or scene as he thinks the worst actor would do it, and then repeat the scene without imposing on it. Usually the actor finds much more freedom and is less afraid to be more expressive. Tina Packer asked me to do this while I was studying at Shakespeare & Company. I was so afraid to be a "bad actor" that I was not committing to anything. Once I had done this exercise, however, I realized the sky did not cave in, and it left me free to experiment without fear.

If the actors sound stilted and do not seem to really be talking to each other:

- Suggest the actors improvise within the situation of the play, and then go back to the actual text. This often makes the actor speak the text more naturally. This can be especially helpful with classical text. It can help to go back and forth a few times between the improvised speaking and the actual text.

If the actor needs help in fully embodying the words and taking ownership of what he is saying:

- In a group context, cast the actor in a high-status role, such as an important movie producer, casting agent, or political figure, and introduce the actor to the group as this very important person; have the group improvise with this in mind and then take the text and see how this informs it.
- Ask the actor to visualize wearing a sound cape, imagining sighing out on a *huh* or *hah* or *hey* sound, thinking of the sound out the imaginary cape. Then repeat this with the thought. In a group, one can ask other actors to hold up the cape, helping to support.
- If the actor is tending to pull down and squeeze the text, one can ask the actor to put on an imaginary crown and give the actor king or queen status. This often helps the actor gain a sense of entitlement to speak and take more ownership of what he is saying.
- Ask the actor(s) to dance as he speaks the text. This is especially useful when actors may intellectually understand the text but physically be stiff with it, constricting the breath. They can simply employ free-form dance or more structured dance movements such as the tango, a waltz, cha-cha, or whatever else the actor may be familiar with. When the actor(s) returns to the text, generally this exploration informs the delivery, allowing for more vocal freedom and a fully kinesthetic connection to the language.
- Have the actor imagine a sound "tutu" and picture the sound coming out of the tutu first on "hah" and then speak the text, imagining the words coming out of the tutu.

If the actor seems to be flattening the natural peaks and valleys of the text and needs to deepen his experience of the rhythm of the language, particularly dealing with iambic pentameter:

- Have the actor sing the text in different styles (country and western, jazz, lounge singer, etc.) and then go back to speaking it. This helps actors find the inherent rhythm of the text, and is especially useful in Shakespeare to explore the iambic pentameter. One might sing the text as an opera or a country and western tune and then speak it. Or one might sing it as a blues number and then speak the text. In a group, one can ask other actors to act as backup singers and sing the operative words to underline these to the actor. Then the actor can speak the text without the backs and see how this informs the delivery.

- Have the actor speak the text, exaggerating the iambic and dancing in that rhythm. If this is done with a group, the other actors may help by tapping out the rhythm. If one has tambourines or even pots and forks, one can do a jazz riff type improvisation with the text and then take the text again without the rhythm. Usually one finds much more liveliness in the delivery. (Ben Benison taught me this exercise at the Royal Academy of Dramatic Art in London.)

- When I was studying with Patsy Rodenburg, she made an important point, which was that when one is exaggerating or even tapping out the iambic, make sure that the second emphasized beat is an upward beat rather than a downward beat. This helps the actor think of the thoughts building on top of each other and moving forward, springboarding into the next thought.

- Take the text as if one is rapping. One actor raps the text and the others can repeat key words as the rapper speaks. Then the actor takes the text again without imposing that on it and generally finds a stronger connection to the rhythm. This is especially good in working with teens and children.

If the actor is tending to push vocally and physically tighten as he speaks the text:

VOICE AND TEXT EXPLORATIONS 119

- Ask the actor to lie on his back, and then speak text, with eyes closed. This helps the actor find the imagery of the language. When the actor is lying on the floor, the shoulders and neck can relax (sometimes the person may need a book under his head if the head is falling back). The actor can experience fuller and easier breathing on the floor. Then when the actor delivers the text standing, hopefully he will maintain some of the ease and relaxation from the floor.

If the actor's jaw is tight in the delivery and the full shape of the words and thoughts are not coming across:

- Suggest the actor take the text with the outline of the tongue resting on the outline of the lower lip, just where the tongue can release and not be fully stretched. Then have the actor speak the text, keeping the tongue on the lower lip. Then slide the tongue back into the mouth and speak the text again. Generally, the jaw is more released and the text is fuller. (I learned this studying with Kristin Linklater.)

- Place clean fingers inside the mouth, gently resting them between the back teeth, and speak the text. Then remove the fingers but keep the same amount of space between the upper and lower back molars and notice that the jaw should be more released.

If an actor is tending to drop final words, then ask him to improvise the following:

- Speak each thought and pass the thought on the final word to someone as if it is a gift or object. You can use a real object if one is available, like a book, a piece of fruit, or a cup. This will help the actor to complete his thought because he is thinking the action through to the end, with the help of the physical action. The actor being given the thought must be careful to really receive fully.

- Ask the actor to mouth the words but only speak the final words, and then go back and speak all the words and notice how the final word has a bit more energy.

One can do this with the first word of a thought if the actor is tending to drop those. Ask the actor to speak the first words and mouth the rest of the thought, and then go back to use all the words and see what he has found. Finally, one can speak the first word of the thought, mouth the thought, and then speak the final word of the thought and then go back and speak the whole thought, saying all the words. This helps the actor clearly book-end the thought at the onset and the completion. Often, when one is coaching a show, one needs to give reminders on clearly starting a thought with the first word and completing the thought with the final word, right to the end of the final consonants, again, so as to springboard into the next thought cleanly. This is a good way to help actors address the tendency to slide into the ideas and drop off the ends of words.

- Have the actors work in partners. Let partner A begin speaking and deliberately trail off in her thought, about ¼ way through. Then A speaks again and extends the thought a bit further, about ½ way through, and then lets it trail off, and so on until the actor has fully completed her thought. B can observe and give feedback to what the actor noticed. Often actors do not realize the mental energy (not to be confused with pushing vocally) required to really complete a thought and let it land fully. Then the actor can take a section of text, paying particular attention to really following the through-line of the complete thought to the absolute end of the last syllable in the last word.

If the actor is monotone:

- Speak the text, exaggerating the pitches, and then speak it.

- Using a piano, take the first line of text on a low pitch, then the next thought a half note higher, and go up in pitch with each new thought. When a full idea is completed, then drop the pitch lower and begin again. The actor can sing this or chant it. Then repeat the text without imposing this and see what one finds.

VOICE AND TEXT EXPLORATIONS

If the actor is tending to blur thoughts:

- Take a prop to represent each new point in an argument. You can pick just about anything. While coaching *The Jew of Malta*, I asked the actors to play out pieces of text with paper clips and pencils to represent each new image, especially when it had to do with a battle or a ship arriving in Cyprus. One can use a bottle of hand lotion as a chess piece and move it on each new thought. Working in pairs, one can have a few props and have the actors play chess on each line—especially useful if it is a competitive scene.

- Put the group into a sculpture. Have an actor speak the text to a different member of the group on each new thought. As the actor speaks a particular thought, the actor wakes up a particular member of the group. This helps the actor identify the thoughts more clearly, generally finding a more committed vocal quality through the process.

- Ask one actor to act as a museum guide. On each new thought within the text, the museum guide introduces a new "exhibit." The other group members follow along with the text and form the image of each new thought just before the actor speaks it. The actor then treats the group as if it is part of an exhibit at a museum and uses the text to describe it. This will help the actor break up the thoughts more specifically, and is particularly useful for someone who rushes over images. It is also a listening exercise for the other actors.

- This is similar to the exercise above. Have the rest of the cast act as a visual aid for the actor. As the actor speaks a particular image, the rest of the cast forms the picture, so the actor can see it as he is saying it. Once the cast has the feeling for their various parts, then take that section of text again, with the cast acting out each new image or event, as the actor speaks. This helps the actor become more specific in his thoughts and gain more awareness of the differentiation of beats within the text.

If the actor isn't able to distinguish images and thoughts and is not using operative words clearly:

- Have two actors take a scene and have the rest of the cast do sound effects like it was a radio play. If the ideas get abstract, one can do a more abstract sound interpretation. This can work particularly well if the actors are off book and can close their eyes as they hear the various sound effects, so they start to differentiate among wind, rain, and the like. Then when they do the scene again, they generally have a livelier and more imaginative relationship to the language and tend to hit the appropriate words in a more organic way.

If the actor needs to develop more contrast between opposites and the conflicts in a piece:

- Have other actors play a good angel and a bad angel, each responding to the actor's text by whispering in the actor's ear after each thought. For example, the good angel might whisper, "It's your fault; you have no right to feel like this" after "What's this? What's this?" "You are perverse to find her attractive." "Is it her fault or mine?" "Of course it's your fault, you are a sinner." And the bad angel might whisper after "Who sins most?": "She is putting a spell on you, she is working on you, of course she's the sinner," and so on, clocking the changes through the speech.

   Angelo's speech, *Act II, scene ii*:

   Angelo:
   What's this, what's this? Is this her fault or mine?
   The tempter or the tempted, who sins most?
   Ha!
   Not she: nor doth she tempt: but it is I
   That, lying by the violet in the sun,
   Do as the carrion does, not as the flower,
   Corrupt with virtuous season. Can it be
   That modesty may more betray our sense
   Than woman's lightness? Having waste ground enough,

> Shall we desire to raze the sanctuary
> And pitch our evils there? O, fie, fie, fie!
> What dost thou, or what art thou, Angelo?
> Dost thou desire her foully for those things
> That make her good? O, let her brother live!
> Thieves for their robbery have authority
> When judges steal themselves. What, do I love her,
> That I desire to hear her speak again,
> And feast upon her eyes? What is't I dream on?
> O cunning enemy, that, to catch a saint,
> With saints dost bait thy hook! Most dangerous
> Is that temptation that doth goad us on
> To sin in loving virtue: never could the strumpet,
> With all her double vigour, art and nature,
> Once stir my temper; but this virtuous maid
> Subdues me quite. Even till now,
> When men were fond, I smiled and wonder'd how.

- Another way to explore this is by switching chairs. For example, in Hamlet's "To be or not to be" speech, one can use a chair for the "to live" part of the monologue and another chair for the "not to live." Each time Hamlet explores the to die idea, the actor sits in the live chair and when Hamlet examines the to live idea, the actor moves to the other chair. One might want to include a third chair to represent the afterlife.

If the actor isn't really getting behind the argument, one can create scenarios based on the text:

- For example, if someone were playing Lady Percy in *Henry IV*, Part II, create a talk show where the topic is "women who have lost their husbands in war, when fathers didn't support them." Have the Lady Percy on one team and her father on the other. Perhaps some fellow fathers can support the father's point of view and Lady Percy can have a support team. The actors have to be careful not get too loud, so as not to drown out the other actors, as people can get a bit excited with this one. Here is a case when one can improvise first and then ask Lady Percy to speak the text again.

If the actor is having trouble getting across the argument of a piece:

- Have the actor use a prop or furniture to represent each new piece of evidence to support the argument. One can use just about anything for this. The actor can place all the evidence in a pile in the middle of the room or build a "map" of the evidence on a table using things like cups, spoons, pencils, or anything. (This exercise is also helpful when the text keeps referring back to something because the actor has to go back to the original prop and thereby realize that the ideas are building on one another.)

- Then the actor takes the text again without the props to see how the exploration informs the text. Generally, the actor finds a more precise connection to the argument and is much clearer.

- The actor takes the text as if she is a lawyer, summing up her final arguments. One can also ask the group to respond with a "hum" when a point hits home.

If the actor is not speaking the words intelligibly, then I would suggest using Cicely Berry's exercise:

- Say the text solely on the consonants but still thinking the thoughts; then solely on the vowels, still thinking the thoughts. When one explores this, it is important to keep the support and release, so as not to tighten in the voice and push from the throat. If the actor is tending to push from the throat, taking the vowels on a yawn to lift the soft palate helps. If the actor is tending to push on the consonants, then massage the tongue root (the soft area underneath the chin); at least it should be soft, but if the muscle is overly tight it will feel sinewy. Then repeat the text, with the vowels and consonants, and notice how this helps shape the thoughts. This exploration also helps the actor connect more with the shape of the language.

If the text is a monologue with some introspection and the actor is experiencing difficulty with the thoughts:

- Have the actor speak the text as if to a therapist, with another actor playing the therapist and asking questions. It can help to begin this as an improvisation and then go on to the text itself. This often helps the actor find the ladder of the thoughts and the events that move the monologue forward.

If the actor is not developing the themes fully:

- One person speaks the text and others repeat words to do with a specific idea or image. For example, the group repeats words to do with love, war, loss, money, negativity, hope, and such. Then the actor goes through the text again, without the group, and generally finds a more specific relationship to words associated with the particular image. It works well to ask the actor or members of the group for suggestions of themes as this gets them more involved in the process.

If the actor is not enunciating clearly:

- Explore consonants and vowels. As the actor speaks the text, the others repeat key consonants. Then the actor speaks the text again without the group to see how this informs the text. Then the actor speaks the text again and the group repeats the vowels. The actor speaks the text again. Generally, this heightens the actor's awareness of the shape of the words and thoughts after this exploration.

- Repeat the consonants exercise: If one does this exercise, make sure the person has never had a stuttering problem. That said, one could ask the person to repeat consonants a few times before going on to the full words. For example, "T-t-t-t-oo b-b-bee or-r-r n-n-n-ot t-t . . . t-t-too b-b-bee . . . " Then go back to the text without the repetition of the consonants and see what one finds.

126   THE THOUGHT PROPELS THE SOUND

If the actor is reciting the text, some of the following explorations can help develop spontaneity:

- Imagine one is speaking the text in a different setting such as a pub or a political rally or gospel revival meeting. This can be done individually or as a group. Break up into groups, where each group approaches the text in a different way: one group does it as a nightclub act crooner à la Frank Sinatra, another does it as a gospel revival, another does rap, and another as if they are in a pub. Then each group presents their exploration, and then repeats the text without the theme approach, and one sees how it has informed the text.

- Lego blocks: Say one word of the text, then stop, then say that word and go on to the next word, stop the thought, then start again from the first word and go onto the next word. For example, "To . . . to be . . . to be or . . . to be or not . . . to be or not to . . . ," then repeat the whole phrase, "To be or not to be." One can get a stronger sense of the build of the thought this way. (I learned this studying with Patsy Rodenburg.)

- Say the text like a melodramatic actor and then repeat it. Often, actors find that some of what they originally perceived as melodramatic really is not.

When an actor is having difficulty adjusting to the theater space after having been in the rehearsal hall:

- Russian doll kinesphere exercise: Think of the Russian dolls that have incrementally smaller dolls nested inside them. Start with the image of the smallest doll and speak a piece of text as if you are that small. Then go to the next sized doll, imagining you are speaking from the sternum to just below your navel. Then imagine you are going to the next sized doll and extend your awareness to include the torso up to the collar bones and speak with this awareness. Then expand your awareness to the next sized doll, thinking of including the jaw down to the midthigh and speak the text. Then imagine going to the next size doll and include from your feet to the top of your head as you speak. Then imagine an even bigger doll, speaking with your sense of kinesphere extending beyond your head and feet and speak the text. Then extend your awareness even further out, make yourself a bigger-than-life doll and speak the text. This is an imaginative way to find how to expand to a bigger playing space by expanding one's kinesthetic awareness, without pushing. It is important in this exercise to keep including the back awareness as one expands into the imaginary dolls.

- Camera angles: One can play with speaking text, after having done the above exercise, imagining expanding in different directions as one speaks the text, as if there are different camera angles on the actor and the actor has to include that angle of his body in his kinesthetic awareness.

- Near-far (inspired by Francis Thomas): In partners, say a line of text with the person close to you, then the person moves slightly farther away, and then a bit farther away again; the partner listening can let the other know when the text is not clear. In general it is not a question of volume as the space increases but of more precise use of consonants and clarity of thought. One can also do this imagining the person moving further and further away.

- Combine a clown or Comedia exercise and then go on to the required text. Imagine people have come from near and far to see the actor. The actor comes to the center of the stage and the other actors sit spread out in the audience *oohing* and *aahing* in anticipation of the actor. Then the actor does the following:
  - Putting the right leg out to the side, the standing leg bent, foot flexed or pointed, as the actor says the text opening the arms into a loose ballet second position but with the elbows slightly bent:

  "Mesdames" to the right,

  "Messieurs" to the left,

  and now in the center with the hand to the heart,

"C'est moi, Harlequin."

The others actors cheer.

- Then the actor takes the Harlequin exercise again and then, after that is completed, says a line of text.

I led the actors at the Birmingham Conservatory for Classical Theatre[4] through this on the Festival stage and it was quite remarkable how their voices centered and became rich and full of ease, particularly notable in the case of the talented Alana Hawley. She released on a rich, fully textured, and confident sound that I had not heard from her before.

If an individual is having difficulty including his back support:

- Lift arms as one allows the breath in, and then speak text as you bring the arms down, but continue to think long in the spine (remember the spine lengthens as we release the breath). This helps open up the back intercostals as the thought is expressed. (Inspired by Francis Thomas, Head of Voice, Bristol Old Vic.)

- Another variation of this I've developed is to ask the actor to put on angel wings and fluff the wings as one is speaking. This also engages the imagination. Recently, I asked a first-year student to add this to her delivery, as she was extremely tight vocally and pushing from the throat with insufficient breath support. As she fluffed her angel feathers, she became much more engaged, her breath became much easier, and her voice freed up considerably, plus she had the opportunity to experience being an angel.

If one is having difficulty getting the voice and thoughts forward, that is, the text is being swallowed:

- Gently chant text into the face around G for women and low G for men, and then speak it.

---

[4]Under the direction of actress and director Martha Henry at the Stratford Shakespeare Festival, Canada.

As a way to get the overall support for the text:

- Speak the text, imagining the sound coming from the back. Then speak the text, imagining the sound out the front of the face. Then speak the text combining these two ideas, thinking the sound out the front of the face and out the back.

SENSE EXPLORATIONS

Coma Exercise

Have partner A pretend to be in a coma as partner B holds A's hand, sensing A's energy and attempting to communicate with that energy nonverbally. Then after about 5 to 10 minutes of this, depending on the group's concentration, have B say a section of text to A, in the hope that the thoughts can penetrate A's coma state. This is an exercise I learned from Bruce Fertman at the Alexander Alliance; we did the nonverbal part and then I added the text component to adapt it to actors.

Soundscape

Have the actor speak the text with his eyes closed. Then the group interprets the images of the text with sound. In some cases, it might be literal sounds, such as the sound of the sea. In other instances, the sound may be more abstract. The actor speaking the text lets the sound wash through him. Then he speaks the text again, without the sound underneath him. Usually the actor finds many more levels in the text.

While coaching at the Stratford Shakespeare Festival Conservatory Program, I asked the group to do this while Ian Lake, a talented young actor, spoke the opening speech of Orsino's. When he spoke it again, without the soundscape, the whole texture of the text deepened and the images and opposites within the text became much clearer. I developed this exercise while leading a Storytelling Voice workshop in Buffalo, New York, for Spin-a-Story. One of the actors was blind, and as I began teaching the workshop, I realized just about every image I used involved visualization, so I thought of this one as a way to help this storytelling find a more visceral connection to the text, and it worked really well.

Five Senses

Read the text and notice which of the senses are being utilized. I often use the first eight lines of Orsino's speech at the beginning of *Twelfth Night* as he overlaps senses in such an imaginative way:

> If music be the food of love, play on,
> Give me excess of it, that, surfeiting,
> The appetite may sicken, and so die.
> That strain again, it had a dying fall:
> O, it came o'er my ear like the sweet sound
> That breathes upon a bank of violets,
> Stealing and giving odour. Enough, no more;
> 'Tis not so sweet now as it was before.

The actors read through the speech and notice which senses Shakespeare uses and how the senses flow one into one another: "Oh it came o'er my ear like the sweet sound that breathes upon a bank of violets." Then they work in partners. One actor is blindfolded, and the other takes the actor to different "sense" stations. One station would have a variety of smells. The second actor guides the blindfolded actor to smell some of the different smells. Then the second actor takes the blindfolded actor to the "taste" station and feeds the blindfolded actor some food such as orange, chocolate, and so on (obviously one wants to check for any allergies before this exploration). Then the actor goes to the "tactile" station and rubs cream on the actor's hand or arm, and guides the actor to touch different textures of material, wood, warm, cold, and such. Then the blindfolded actor is taken to the "sound" station and listens to some music on CD or piano, or some other sounds, perhaps pleasant and then less pleasant. If possible, it is great to go outside and sense how the air feels different than inside. Then the actors take off the blindfolds and look around. Ideally it is great to have a nice view of something to see. Having been blindfolded and having the other senses stimulated, it can prove quite a delight to experience seeing again. Then the actor who was blindfolded speaks the text again to see if there is more connection to the sensuality of the words within the text. Then the partners switch roles. This can be applied to other texts as well and is particularly useful for exploring Shakespeare.

Summary

The goal of voice and text explorations is to help the actor embody the language and stimulate the imagination. The director might want to include these sorts of explorations with the full cast of a play or use them to help free up particular scenes that may be more challenging in this regard. One finds as one develops these, new ideas occur to suit particular cast needs, and cast members themselves start to offer up ideas. These explorations help deepen the voice and text work and help to build an ensemble in rehearsal.

Explorations along these lines generally work best early on in the rehearsal, while the actors are open to incorporating new information and things have not become too set. As the show gets closer to opening, it is more difficult for actors to integrate new ideas, but something like dancing the text or singing the text might prove a good way to loosen people up.

It is important not to become too result oriented with this kind of work. Sometimes an exercise really helps one actor free up and find something new to the character, but other times—for whatever reason—some exercises may just not gel. A good way to frame things at the onset is to present these explorations with a "take what you like and leave the rest" attitude. An exercise that does not seem to work might stimulate an idea that is extremely useful, so it is important for the director and cast to keep an open mind and commit fully to each exploration with a sense of discovery and playfulness. Even if an idea sounds silly, try it anyway. As a director, it's a good idea to stay open to suggestions from the cast, the vocal coach, or Alexander coach, even when a suggestion may not initially appear particularly helpful. It might work and even if it doesn't, it creates an attitude of experimentation and helps ease the overall anxiety of the production. If there is an inclusive atmosphere in the rehearsal hall, this will help the overall ensemble feeling, which is important to establish at the onset of rehearsals and enhances the overall production.

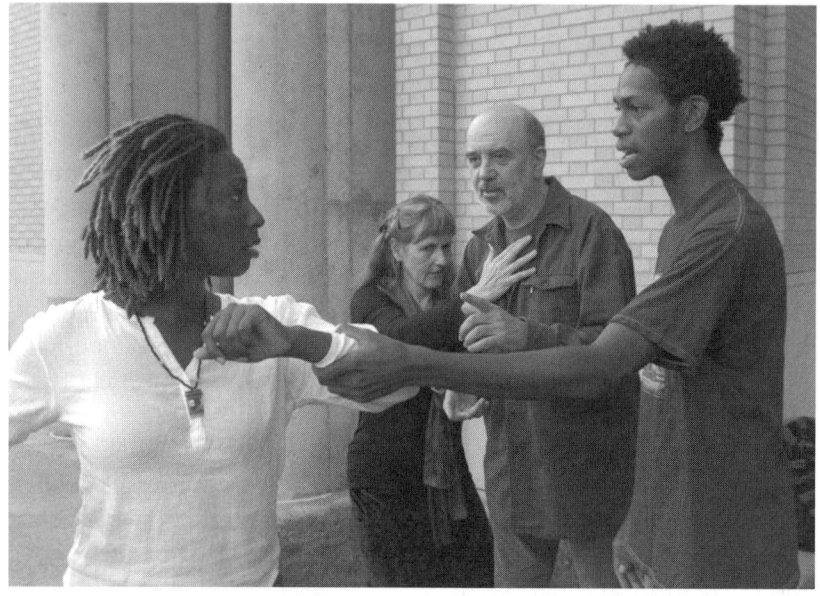

Left to right, Roberta Burke (BFA, Acting, School of Drama, Carnegie Mellon, 2009), Janet Madelle Feindel (author), Mladen Kiselov (director), and Eric Berryman (BFA, Acting student, School of Drama, Carnegie Mellon). Photo by Karen Waggoner.

CHAPTER 8

Directors, Voice, and the Rehearsal Process

SUPPORTING THE VOCAL PROCESS WITH TEXT WORK

The director supports healthy voice usage by giving actors a thorough and detailed textual analysis of the play. The director must understand the build of thoughts and how characters affect each other. It is extremely important not to take text analysis for granted but rather to break down each scene in specific detail. If the director does not grasp the details, how can she expect the actors to? Directing training programs often place a great deal of emphasis on "conceptualizing" the play at the expense of a thorough grasp of the structure of the play. When this is the case, actors are less likely to breathe in a way that connects the breath organically to the thought. They tend not to articulate clearly because they do not entirely understand what they are saying or why. Without a solid foundation in the text, actors push for emotion and effect, which unfortunately separates them from the real intention of the character. Vocal strain often results in such a situation.

GIVING ACTING NOTES TO SUPPORT HEALTHY VOICE USAGE

As outlined earlier, directors can help actors achieve proper voice usage by giving specific action notes rather than "state of being" notes. More specifically, it is most useful to suggest to an actor "something to do" rather than something to feel or "be." If the scene involves anger, rather than saying, "You're angry" or "Get angry," the director helps the actor more if she suggests, "Really attack her here" or "Rub her nose in that"; the more volatile the suggestion, the better. As outlined in *A Practical Handbook for the Actor* (Bruder et al., 1986), the director should make the note "hot." For example, an actor with an objective like "I want to help her out of a bad situation" should think in a more explosive fashion: "I am saving her from a disaster." Recently, I coached a student production of *The Three Sisters*. The actor playing Koolyghin came to me for a tutorial session. I asked what his intention was in his first scene. He said, "I am giving Irina a birthday present." I asked, "And why?" "Well, it is her birthday." "Is there a deeper reason you might be giving her a birthday present?" "What do you mean?" he asked. "For example, if you give her a birthday present as a symbol of your love it might make the memory of her father's death less painful, might please Masha and make her easier to live with, and this may improve your marriage, which isn't doing all that great, or—conversely—it might make Masha a bit jealous, so she will pay you more attention. This might improve your life together and give your own life more meaning and joy." Get the picture? I am pleased to say he took the suggestion and applied the same principle to other scenes as well and his performance improved enormously. Had he begun from a deeper exploration of the intention, however, he would have been able to delve that much more deeply into the character at the onset of rehearsals, or even before they had begun. When the objective is superficial, the voice work is as well. When the actor's attention is on affecting someone else, the voice is far more supported, with a clear forward tone. The intention propels the sound forward in an organic way.

Often I have asked a student actor (and sometimes professional actors as well), "What is your intention?" and the actor tells me, "Well, I am angry" or some other state of being. Again, when an actor goes for an emotional state, she tends to push vocally. She puts her attention on the end result rather than on communication with another person. She monitors the emotion rather than monitoring whether or not her character successfully achieves her goal. This renders the actor self-conscious, and self-consciousness is the enemy of good acting.

An experienced actor recounted the following incident in rehearsal for a production of *Uncle Vanya*, directed by a well-respected European director. He told the actor playing the professor, "You really lose it there." The actor told me: "I became so concerned with losing it, that I ended up just yelling, rather than playing my intention because I wanted to please the director. After the scene, I realized that I had pushed my voice and felt hoarse—and silly." I suggested doing a quick mental adjustment of the note. Rather than thinking of "losing it," he might think of "leveling" the people he's onstage with, or "setting them straight." The director's note may well have accurately described where the character should end up, but not the *process* for getting there. The responsibility for achieving what the director suggests ultimately belongs to the actor. It helps enormously, however, if the director makes that extra effort to guide the actor as specifically as possible, particularly in scenes involving high intensity where the risk of vocal strain is greater.

When I was working on the character Blanche in scene 10 in Tennessee Williams' *A Streetcar Named Desire*, as described in Chapter 7, Voice and Text Explorations, the process was much more effective than if Berry had said, "Play the scene angry."

In using a physical activity as a metaphor for the character's struggle, I connected to the inner workings of the character, which enabled the full range of vocal expression. Certainly, the anger welled up inside me, but I put my attention on pushing him away both literally and figuratively. I depended on the language to shape the scene. Had I simply attempted to portray anger, I would have become superficial, self-conscious, and vocally tight. It also spurred me on to avoid the pitfall of playing Blanche as the "crazy" victim rather than a woman fighting for survival—a much more engaging choice. The exercise also gave the actor playing Stanley a focus and fed the power struggle between the two characters. This exploration enabled us to eschew the tendency to simply "yell" at each other with no real build to the scene.

Blanche does not deliberately act crazy; she desperately wants to achieve a normal life, whatever that means to her. The obstacles to attaining that life may well drive her crazy, but that does not mean she needs to play crazy. She needs to go after the life she wants as vigorously as she can: by getting Mitch to marry her, by contacting Shep Huntley, and so on. Moving the actions of the character forward allows the actor playing her to connect the breath in a fuller manner so the voice reveal the nuances of the character's struggle. Michael Shurtleff reminds the reader in *Audition* (2003) with this example: Chekhov's *Three Sisters* is not a play about three sisters who never make it to Moscow, but a play about three sisters who fight to get there.

When the actor chooses a positive, active intention and uses the voice and language to communicate that intention, the voice can then become lively and full. Clearly, the actor's overall instrument must also be properly tuned, and she needs to understand the mechanics of healthy voice usage: proper breath support, clear diction, and use of forward resonance. The final step of developing a strong performance integrated with good voice usage involves what Shurtleff (2003) calls "interfering" with your partner. The actor's motivational process and the manner in which the voice reveals the nuances of character are intrinsically linked.

Sensitivity to Actors

When a director rehearses an intense scene, it helps to take frequent breaks, so as not to overtire the actors. During rehearsals, actors may rehearse a scene over and over, out of context of the entire play, and thus increase the risk of vocal pushing. Actors are often poor about warming up before rehearsals, whereas they will likely warm up before an actual performance. As a result, the director needs to emphasize warm-ups before rehearsals, especially in preparation for intense or climactic scenes. Directors help actors by showing sensitivity to scene content. A few years ago, a student actress came to me for a tutorial, quite upset because she had rehearsed a rape scene 10 times the night before. No doubt the director felt this repetition contributed to the sense of reality to the scene, but the actress herself felt violated. The men in the scene also reported in tutorials that the frequent repetition of the rape scene was disturbing beyond what they felt was useful for the play. It is important in such situations for the director to stop and frame the scene, take a break, and discuss what is happening, particularly with student actors. One must remember with less experienced actors not to underestimate the intimidation factor, even when one is not a particularly intimidating person. Just being in a position of authority, which directors are, can be intimidating (and this is doubled if the director is also one's teacher). Although this example may not seem specifically related to voice, the reality is that one cannot separate the emotional state of the actor from voice production. The actor's vocal release must remain free, with full breath support, even in a high-intensity scene. If the emotional content is extremely intense and the actor, not the character, is uncomfortable, this will inevitably affect the actor's physical ease and hence the voice use. The actor must feel emotional support and respect from the director offstage to successfully achieve the necessary freedom on stage. It behooves the director to think of directing as a collaborative process and check in often with the actors to see how they are dealing with challenging content. Of course, a voice and Alexander coach can offer enormous support in these situations as well.

Growth of the scene can also be compromised with repeated rehearsals of emotionally disturbing scenes. Rehearsing such scenes more than three or four times may create tension for the actor, which often manifests as muscle tightness around the larynx and other areas of the vocal apparatus. This sort of physical strain makes the actor more susceptible to vocal damage. Although some directors may think repetition or actually disturbing the actor as a person adds to the development and "the truth" of a scene, in some cases the potential psychological and vocal costs to the actor are too high. The director should consult with actors as well as give them time to process the scene. Directors do not have the license to abuse actors physically or emotionally, nor do voice coaches. Actors have an obligation to express concerns regarding anything in rehearsal that may be causing them physical and/or emotional harm. Any reasonable director should take those concerns seriously. Of course, by the same token, actors do not have the right to verbally abuse directors, other actors, voice or Alexander coaches, or stage management. Sometimes actors take advantage of powerful positions and create havoc in rehearsals. Obviously, this is hardly helpful to the overall process.

VOCAL PREPARATION (WARM-UPS)

At the first read-through, a director should emphasize the importance of healthy vocal use, stressing the importance of a daily warm-up. If the director is qualified to lead a warm-up, she can lead a simple Vox Explora, as outlined in Chapter 5. Otherwise, she can assign a cast member with the appropriate training to lead warm-ups. Certainly, actors graduating from Carnegie Mellon and most major drama schools should have the ability to lead a safe, basic warm-up. In general, actors trained in the work of Fitzmaurice, Smukler, Linklater, Berry, Wade, and/or Rodenburg should be able to lead a solid vocal warm-up. Ideally, the director or stage manager should arrange for the person to receive credit on the program as voice captain.

The director should allot time within the rehearsal process for warm-ups. These warm-ups should be a minimum of 15 minutes to accomplish the task, with 20 to 30 minutes even better. Warm-ups are especially important before full run-through of acts and of the full play. Not only does this activity help actors' vocal use, it helps to build a stronger company ensemble. This sense of ensemble enables the actors to communicate the nuances of the play with greater sensitivity. If the cast includes any established actors, their involvement in and support of the warm-up is important. The younger actors learn by example that the practice of voice technique is ongoing throughout one's career. It may prove difficult to schedule warm-ups on days when calls involve staggered rehearsal times for the actors. Nonetheless, the director can certainly stress that actors should come to rehearsals prepared vocally—even if the actor must warm up on her own time. The director's support of the warm-ups will pay dividends in terms of the quality of the voices and the sense of ensemble, and hence the overall quality of the production.

During the artistic directorship of Robin Phillips at the Stratford Festival, daily warm-ups were part of the acting company's call, and the leading actors of the company participated in the warm-ups. Participation by actors like Brian Bedford, Maggie Smith, Martha Henry, Richard Monette, and Nicholas Pennell provided an excellent example for the younger company members. This attention to vocal preparation was evident in the high level of vocal quality of the shows at the time.

While coaching (alongside Cicely Berry) for Theatre for a New Audience's *The Jew of Malta* (directed by David Herskovits) and *The Merchant of Venice* (directed by Darko Tresnjak) (performed in repertory with the same cast), I led warm-ups before all the previews and opening shows, and then Kate Forbes took over as voice captain after opening night. It took a bit of negotiation but, due to

Jeffrey Horowitz's efforts on the cast's behalf, we were able to do the warm-up on the stage, which was enormously helpful to the actors. In most cases in the United States, one has to make the warm-up voluntary. With the Theatre for a New Audience shows, almost all the cast participated in the warm-up and it made a huge difference to the quality of the production. When the show moved to England as part of the Royal Shakespeare's Complete Works Festival, the TFANA cast participated in the RSC warm-ups, and this was really exciting for them. At the RSC, all the cast members attend the warm-ups, from the likes of Ian McKellen to a beginning journeyman. The company's voice work grew even stronger in the United Kingdom than it had been in New York, which I attribute in large part to the extended work they did with Cicely Berry and the group warm-ups with the full RSC company. The vitality of the language and the vocal interaction between characters was electric and palpable. I nearly jumped up on the stage and shook Antonio (played by Tom Nellis) in the first act for not having accepted Shylock's (played by F. Murray Abraham) attempt at reconciliation—and this was after having seen the show at least 30 times! I completely forgot I was watching two actors whom I had worked with for many weeks, and was completely absorbed in the characters.

VOCAL HEALTH

Within a rehearsal process, a number of pitfalls exist in which vocal stress and strain can occur. As discussed above, during rehearsals actors may repeat a demanding scene over and over without the full arc to the play to support the scene's intensity. The air in rehearsal halls may be dry from air conditioning or overheating, which can create vocal difficulties for the actor. The stress of the insecure nature of the actor's lifestyle can also create a certain tension. Perhaps an actor has not worked for some months prior to this engagement or the actor has not worked with this particular director before. The actor may attempt to do everything "right." This may cause an overall tension in the actor's delivery, resulting in vocal strain. The actor may hold a day job or need to audition for other roles during the rehearsal period or length of the run. Actors often work on readings, voice-overs, and commercials during the course of a run. All of these activities can create a situation in which the actor can become tense. In short, many factors exist to interfere with healthy voice usage.

Vocal Injuries

Many individuals can develop vocal fatigue from overuse, a cold, exposure to dust, flu, or a number of other reasons. In most cases, with adequate fluids and rest, the voice returns to healthy use in a few days.

If there is a coach working on the show, it is a good idea for the director or stage management to consult with the coach, as she may be able to help or steer the actor to someone who can help. When I was coaching at the Stratford Festival, a talented actor, Benedict Campbell. was playing Duncan in *Macbeth*. He had a bad cold and was rather hoarse, making it difficult for him to say his lines. The stage management was about to call an understudy rehearsal when I happened to walk into the stage management office. I said, "I know it's a novel concept, but why not consult with the voice coach first?" They laughed and I said, "Give me Ben for 40 minutes and I will see what I can do." I worked with him, using some methods for voice restoration I learned from Kristin Linklater during my teacher training with her. He was able to regain about 80% of his voice back. Not perfect, of course, but good enough to perform that evening, provided he rested his voice the rest of the time. The theater, the actor, and the understudy were spared unnecessary stress and concern. So, when in doubt, consult the vocal coach as she may be able to help!

It is great if the theater staff can develop a relationship with medical experts who specialize in professional voice users. The ideal is an interdisciplinary clinic that includes laryngologists, speech pathologists, speaking voice teachers, singing teachers, Alexander teachers, psychologists, and other specialists focusing on the professional voice user. One such example is the American Institute for Voice and Ear Research in Philadelphia, under the direction of Robert Sataloff, MD, DMA, FACS. The interdisciplinary approach provides a multileveled course of action to the complex care that the professional voice user requires. As mentioned in the Preface, many such interdisciplinary clinics exist in major cities (see Resources at the end of the book.)

Voice injuries can vary greatly in terms of gravity as well as the long- or short-term impact on performance. If an actor becomes hoarse, there can be a multitude of reasons. Generally, hoarseness should not last more than a few days, and if it does, it is important to have it checked with a reputable medical doctor who specializes in professional voice users. The rule of thumb is, when in doubt, one should see a doctor and receive a laryngeal "scope" to determine any medical issues that may need treatment. Maladies such as reflux or allergies are easily diagnosed and, generally, easily treated. If left untreated, however, reflux, for example, may cause more serious medical conditions. Other issues, such as nodules and polyps, often require more ongoing medical treatment and voice therapy. On the more serious end of the spectrum, some prolonged hoarseness may indicate a life-threatening issue such as laryngeal cancer, which requires immediate and complex treatment. Actors sometimes will attempt various home remedies that can complicate rather than solve the problem, but it's important to get a sound diagnosis in order to get the most effective treatment.

Actors should let doctors know if they are taking medications, including serotonin inhibitors, tranquilizers, and—what many actors do not realize—any herbal treatments, as these may be contraindicated with certain more traditional medical treatments.

Whatever the vocal issue, rest, proper hydration (that is, drinking plenty of water), and, wherever possible, a properly humidified environment are of great help.

Some Basic Tips

Actors need regular vocal rests. Normally, equity breaks are scheduled every 90 minutes. When an actor exhibits vocal fatigue (hoarseness, crackling sound in the voice when the actor shifts registers, etc.), the director does well to take more frequent breaks than the equity requirements.

If an actor develops hoarseness, she should not whisper. This is more harmful for the voice than normal speaking. The director should make sure there's plenty of drinking water available in rehearsal halls. If the hall is unusually dry (unfortunately, most are), the director may insist on a vaporizer or humidifier.

The director (or stage manager) should be aware of a nearby physician specializing in voice care for performers, usually a local otolaryngologist if a voice coach is not available. Some major cities house voice clinics, which are staffed by interdisciplinary teams of otolaryngologists, ear/nose/throat specialists (ENTs), voice teachers, singing teachers, Alexander teachers, and speech pathologists dedicated to the care and treatment of the professional voice user. These professionals should be well trained to help in a vocal emergency. Ideally, a director might make contact with them ahead of rehearsals, to establish a working relationship. Then appropriate professionals are already aware of the production in the unfortunate event of a vocal emergency.

In Philadelphia, Dr. Robert Sataloff's interdisciplinary team includes Mary J. Hawkshaw and Margaret Baroody, MM, and works closely with both singers and actors in the area and internationally. In the Toronto area, the administrations of a number of theater companies such as the Stratford Festival, the Canadian Opera Company, and the Royal Alexandra Theatre have built an ongoing relationship with Vox Cura, an interdisciplinary team of voice care professionals led by Dr. Brian Hands. In Pittsburgh, the University of Pittsburgh houses an interdisciplinary voice clinic led by Clark Rosen, MD, and including the gifted Katherine Verdolini, PhD, and Rita Hersan, MA, SLP. In New York, Gwen Korovin, MD, works with the Gould Center for the Care of the Voice, and Peak Woo, MD, is director of the Eugene Grabscheid Voice Center. Further information about similar clinics can be obtained from the Voice Foundation. (See Resources.) If an actor does receive emergency treatment, a thank-you to the individual staff member involved and the name of the clinic in the theater program with a couple of complimentary tickets are a welcome professional courtesy.

USE OF DIALECTS AND ACCENTS

Most people use the term *dialect coach* or *dialect consultant* and assume the person coaches accents as well, which generally they do. A *dialect*, however, actually refers to variations of sounds and rhythms of native speech. A person whose mother tongue is English might speak with an Irish, New York, Newfoundland, or Cockney dialect. For example, Gwyneth Paltrow uses a Standard British dialect (excellently coached by Barbara Berkery) in *Shakespeare in Love*, but her own dialect is General American. Daniel Day Lewis uses an American dialect in his work in the film *The Age of Innocence*. An *accent* refers to the sounds and rhythms that influence a speaker when the language spoken is other than the speaker's mother tongue. For example, Gérard Depardieu in the film *Green Card* uses a French accent while speaking English. If he were speaking French, he would use some dialect of French. Of course, the dialect of the character's native tongue can subtly influence the accent in another language. A Sicilian speaking English would sound slightly different than a Roman speaking English.

Every dialect and accent has a set of sound changes that occur. Phonetic symbols or simpler dictionary symbols can be used to denote these sounds, much as one uses notation to depict particular notes in music. The actor can learn the sound changes and place the symbol as a reminder on her script. Rhythm changes also occur; for example, some dialects and accents tend to inflect upward in pitch at the end of a line and others downward. Some have more musicality than others. Standard British often inflects up at the end of the thought, whereas General American usually inflects down, and Irish dialects tend to be more musical than North American dialects. Actors can utilize symbols for these changes as well.

Most actors learn dialects and accents through a combination of hearing the sound and rhythm changes and learning them from other sources. Each coach and/or actor develops her own approach, usually based on a variety of methods available. What is most important in learning an accent or dialect is that the accent or dialect does not dominate the acting. The actor must always play the intention, not the dialect or accent. The accent or dialect can often obscure meaning if this is not tended to with special attention. Once the dialect or accent is mastered, the actor needs to put extra attention on clarity and intention. If the dialect or accent is so thick that the clarity is lost, even if it is authentic, it is best to pull back on the accent or dialect, rather than risk losing the text altogether. One may have to take some dramatic license in certain dialects such as Cockney, which to a North American ear particularly can be difficult to understand. There is nothing more tedious than watching an actor "play the dialect" instead of the scene.

There exist numerous methods for attaining dialects and accents if a coach is not available. These include audio selections on CDs, a variety of Web sites through the Voice and Speech Trainers

Association (VASTA), and films set in the appropriate region. In some cases, a CD only includes examples of the dialect or accent played by the coach, which tend to be less accurate and less effective as learning tools. One needs to augment these with examples of native speakers. Some approaches are better for North Americans and some are better for Europeans, so the coach and actor will do well to shop around for the most accurate sources and guides for each particular dialect. (See Resources.)

The following advice may sound strange coming from a dialect coach, but dialects are best avoided unless integral to the script, particularly when the theater hasn't included a dialect coach's salary in the budget. I saw the touring production of *Equus* at the Place Des Arts in Montreal a number of years ago. Everyone except the boy playing Alan used a British dialect. This threw me initially, but then the production so affected me that I forgot about this inconsistency. My guess is that the dialect interfered with the young actor's performance, and the director told him to drop it. The production did not suffer as a result.

I taught a scene study course at Kent State University involving scenes written by George Bernard Shaw. The American students did not have a background in the British dialect. In their attempts to use it, the dialect was getting in the way of their acting so much that I finally told them not to use it. The actors really connected to the thought process with full commitment, and the lack of dialect did not hurt at all. In fact, it improved the scenes immensely. This would probably not work for an Oscar Wilde script, but for the vigor of the Shaw scenes, it worked surprisingly well.

Many good actors simply are poor at dialects, even with an excellent dialect coach. Timothy Monich, one of the world's most respected dialect coaches, was the dialect coach on the movie *A Dry White Season*, starring the late Marlon Brando. He recounted the following incident. Mr. Monich addressed Marlon Brando and said, "Mr. Brando, the accent you are using sounds more British than South African." Mr. Brando reportedly turned to the director and said, "Make the character British." The director agreed. Brando did not master that dialect either. This dialect flaw, however, did not destroy the performance of this talented actor or in any way reflect on the talent of the coach.[1]

---

[1]Conversation at the Department of Drama, University of Alberta, Edmonton, Alberta, 1990.

If the play, in the director's opinion, requires a dialect and/or accent, less is more; that is, the "flavor" of the dialect works most successfully with particular attention to the rhythm of the dialect. Some actors tend to become extremely technical doing dialects, resulting in a stilted quality. They become so focused on making the right sounds that they become self-conscious, which creates a "paint by numbers" quality to the work, and obviously one wants to avoid this at all costs. The real task involves conveying the need of the character through language and ensuring that the dialect serves as an enhancement to the characterization. We shouldn't be overly aware of the dialect. Often when coaching a dialect, the task involves guiding the actors to do less. Actors often introduce more sound changes than actually exist in the dialect, especially in the Standard British dialect. When I coached in Canada, the actors generally mastered the British dialect more quickly than their American counterparts, probably because there are so many British people in Canada that actors have heard the dialect on a regular basis and it is easier to reproduce. My experience in the United States, on the other hand, is that actors master the Irish dialect in a snap. In teaching the Irish dialect, I was using text from the role of Minnie Powell in Sean O'Casey's *Shadow of a Gunman*. The actress found the dialect difficult until I suggested that the sentiments being expressed were not unlike those of the motivation for the American Revolution and, lo and behold, she mastered the dialect beautifully. One must never underestimate the psychological connection to the work. Many times as a coach, one needs to find the best hook for that individual and understand that everyone is different in this regard, which makes the work continually fascinating.

Actors using a dialect or accent often attempt to create the sound by focusing in the throat and mouth area, forgetting to incorporate proper breath support. This mistaken focus contributes to the stiff quality actors often exhibit doing dialect and accents. Actors should explore the physical connection when incorporating a dialect or accent. The director might suggest that the actor dance or sing the scene, or do another physical activity such as running or playing the scene as if it is a tennis match. (See Chapter 7 on Voice and Text Explorations for other ideas.) This helps the actor integrate the dialect in a more believable manner. Actors have a tendency to allow a dialect to limit their vocal range rather than open up their vocal range, so anything that encourages more physical and vocal freedom is always helpful. The director can use dance styles of the appropriate region or historical period as improvisational tools as well. The aim is not to exhaust the actors with such exercises, but to develop a stronger physical connection to the language as the actor incorporates the technical aspects of the dialect or accent.

If the play requires a dialect or accent, the director should encourage the actors to use it early in the rehearsal period so they can incorporate it successfully into the performances. Ideally, actors should begin the study of the dialect several weeks before rehearsal begins. Timothy Monich told me he didn't use phonetics a great deal, as many actors were not familiar with the phonetic alphabet, but he encouraged actors to listen to the dialect or accent for a couple of weeks before even attempting it. That way the actor really gets the dialect into her ear and subconscious.

When I coached British actor Brian Bedford in preparation for an American dialect for his role in the film *Nixon*, I painstakingly prepared phonetic sheets of sound changes from the British to the American dialect. When I presented them to Bedford at our first session, he said, "I don't know phonetics!" I had to think fast on my feet and figure out another way to teach him the sound changes. He had an excellent ear and was able to reproduce them by listening to me say the sounds, though not all actors can master this so easily. If an actor is not able to distinguish and reproduce the sound changes, then the coach can use dictionary symbols or employ a more kinesthetic approach, for example, helping the actor to feel where the placement is in her mouth, where the areas of most resonance are, and so on. The American dialect tends to resonate more in the middle of the mouth, whereas the British and many European dialects tend to resonate more in the front of the mouth. For example, when actors speak using a British dialect, they need to pay attention to the precision of consonants and avoid eliding words. The warm-up exercises that can help the actor accomplish this include the Ybuzz, the teeth resonators and the sinus resonators, and articulating with crisp consonants while maintaining vocal ease so the dialect does not sound forced.

Directors need to emphasize the importance of not playing the dialect but playing the intention, with clarity of the text paramount. Sometimes the text conveys the rhythm of the dialect and accent as well; the actor can simply relax a little, and the dialect begins to happen instinctively. An actor performing Tennessee

Williams' plays, set in the southern United States often finds if he releases the jaw and slows down, that the southern dialect develops quite naturally, simply by surrendering to the rhythm of the language. Even if one spoke Oscar Wilde text with an American accent, an actor with any instinct at all would likely end up speaking with more of a British lift because the text dictates it.

Actors must make the dialect and/or accent intelligible. But if the director must choose between a good performance and a good dialect or accent, the director should choose the performance. However, one hopes to achieve both if possible. When an actor like Daniel Day Lewis integrates a flawless dialect with a masterful performance as he did in the film *In the Name of the Father*, fully incorporating the principles of healthy, expressive voice usage, this is exhilarating for the audience.

SUMMARY

When a director shows sensitivity to healthy voice usage and incorporates this into the rehearsal and performance process, she greatly increases the chance of a more artistically satisfying and successful production. And what director doesn't want that?

CHAPTER 9

Special Issues

*T*here are a number of areas that pose special challenges for actors, coaches, and directors in terms of the voice. Some of these are evident before rehearsals begin, so one has a bit more time to deal with them. However, a number of these challenges appear only during technical rehearsals and can throw the actor off balance. This is where the sensitivity of the director can make a huge difference to the sense of confidence with which the actor goes into opening week.

USE OF FOG AND SMOKE, OR PRESENCE OF DUST IN THE THEATER

During performance, directors do well to eschew special effects like fog or smoke, unless absolutely necessary, because these can cause considerable irritation to actors' vocal apparatus. Equity now has some guidelines regarding the use of specific types of fog or smoke, as some are more actor-friendly than others. These are updated regularly and actors and directors should familiarize themselves with these guidelines. If the director feels the fog or smoke is imperative to the success of the show, he should instruct the technical staff to use as little as possible and direct the smoke at the actors' feet rather than at their faces. If smoke or fog is utilized, the stage management should provide water at a convenient spot either onstage or just offstage within easy access. Most theaters are filled with years of dust and are not well ventilated. All of these factors can serve to irritate the performer's voice. If the director's influence carries any weight at a particular theater, he can suggest proper ventilation and maintaining a level of cleanliness in the theater, paying close attention to things like curtains or furniture, where dust can accumulate. It also helps to have vaporizers available for each dressing room, especially during the dry winter months. Artistic directors can insist on these things.

Sound Cue Levels

An actor's voice is not designed to compete with loud sound cues, particularly if the performers are not using microphones. A good sound designer considers the actor's voice as part of the sound design, although obviously a more spontaneous and lively component. At different points of the play, the design team (including the voice coach) emphasizes specific aspects of the play. The sound design should highlight themes within the play without obscuring important interactions of the actors and significant moments in the text. In general, one wants to avoid sound cues under the actors' speaking unless absolutely necessary to move the plot of the play forward. Most actors will push vocally to compete with loud sound effects. This competition creates a situation in which vocal damage of some kind (such as inflammation of the vocal folds, nodules, or worse, hemorrhaging) can occur. If a sound cue is essential and/or the speaking of the text is secondary at that point, then the actor should not push to compete with the sound cue. In a show I was coaching in New York off Broadway, one of the sound cues was deafening and the actor (who has an especially rich voice), was pushing vocally over the sound cue. The cue obscured the text, which was a fairly important plot point. I spoke to the director, a lovely man but completely unaware on this issue. He said, "But it is such an amazing sound cue." I said, "But you can't understand the wonderful text—the plot point—and this brilliant actor is pushing vocally to speak over the cue and we still can't hear it." I tried several times to have the cue adjusted but it never was. It was quite near opening night and I was concerned if I gave a note directly to the actor that the actor would panic. It was disappointing that this director was more concerned with a sound cue than the actor's performance or the actor's vocal health. People confuse theater with movies. In movies, in most cases, the sound cue comes after the scene is taped, so the actor is not competing with it. Actors should not compete with sound in the theater either, and the fewer sound cues under an actor's text, the better.

A few years ago, I saw a student-directed production of Shakespeare's *The Tempest*. Near the top of the show, the director used thunder sound effects intermittently throughout the storm scene. The level of the sound cue completely drowned out the actors, who attempted, unsuccessfully, to shout over the deafening noise. This annoyed audience members, many of whom complained at intermission and some of whom actually left at intermission. It obscured most of the plot line of the scene, not to mention potentially damaging the actors' voices as well as the actors' and the audience's hearing. Audiences accept a certain amount of dramatic license. The sound level did not need to replicate an actual thunderstorm; a few thunderclaps convey the idea. The director needs to adjust the sound levels so actors don't have to compete with sound effects. If a director feels a sound effect absolutely must be played at maximum volume, then he should provide microphones for the actors, or tape the actors and play the tape at the same time as the sound cue. The sound technicians can adjust the levels so the text remains audible. Sometimes sound designers use dangerously loud sound levels. Again, no one needs to attend the theater (or movies) at the risk of damaging his hearing. Directors need to practice sensitivity in this area, and explore subtler choices and insist the sound designer follow suit. Alternatively, when gunshots or other loud sound cues are included in the sound design, the theater staff should include a sign in the lobby and inform individuals when they are purchasing tickets that this is the case, as is customary with the use of strobe lighting or artificial fog or smoke.

When I coached at the Stratford Festival, I was fortunate that the sound technicians working on the production of *The Boyfriend* were used to working closely with the voice department. In this situation, the sound technicians sought out the input of the voice/dialect coach for advice in how to balance the clarity of the text and lyrics of the songs with the sound levels. This was enormously helpful to the director, musical director, and the actors.

152   THE THOUGHT PROPELS THE SOUND

Unless the play stipulates the sound cue or music cue (such as the Varsuviana sequence in *A Streetcar Named Desire*), acting over background noise or music distracts both actors and audiences. Sounds and music may prove effective in movies because movies are visual, whereas the stage is language-based. We need to let the natural beauty of the solitary human voice reveal the truth of the play. Hitting the audience over the head by underlining scenes with unnecessary, distracting sound or music cues underestimates the intelligence and imagination of the audience.

Use of Microphones

The author wishes to thank Joseph Pino, Assistant Professor of Sound Design, School of Drama, Carnegie Mellon University, for his insights regarding microphone use.

Microphones in the theater are usually used to create a special effect or "vocal close-up," as it were. Sometimes actors take too much for granted when using a microphone; that is, they will become sloppy with clarity, particularly with final consonants or "edges" of words, and sometimes speak more softly than usual. Joseph Pino spoke to the musical theater students I teach at Carnegie Mellon about this phenomenon as "garbage in, garbage out," because the microphone only amplifies what it receives, especially in a live performance. The actor must commit with as much vigilance to the clarity of the thought as he would without the microphone, and think of the microphone only as an enhancement of what he is already doing in the performance. Performers and directors should communicate clearly about why the actor is using the microphone so the actor can adjust his performance accordingly and maintain the full natural release of the voice as opposed to putting on some kind of affectation in the delivery. The microphone often overamplifies sounds such as plosive *b* and *p*, and *s* sounds, so the actor needs to be trained in how to use a microphone in order, for example, to minimize these sounds so that they don't "pop," creating distracting reverberation. The actor should also know how to adjust various types of microphones.

Outdoor productions and some bigger Broadway shows often use "foot mikes," which provide a general boost to the sound and can be adjusted to roll out frequencies of lower than 100 Hz, which is well below even a low-pitched speaking voice. In my experience, however, this general miking is acceptable for outdoors, but for an indoor theater often flattens the nuance of the sound and speaking of text. Well-trained actors should be able to fill an acoustically well-designed space without amplification, with far preferable results. If any microphone is used, the best ones—often used for musicals—are attached to the head with a piece that comes around to the side of the mouth, which remains fixed no matter where the actor moves. This then allows a consistent amplification, though often performers find these headpiece microphones distracting and they are visible to the audience.

The Ambient Sound of Lighting, Heating, and Cooling Equipment

The author wishes to thank lighting designer Allen Hahn for his contribution to the lighting equipment portion of this section.

This section on ambient sounds, caused by some of the new lighting equipment being used in theaters, is based on a discussion I had with Alec Cooper, Master Electrician at the Festival Theatre, Stratford Shakespeare Festival. Cooper, who has worked at the Festival for several decades, constantly refines solutions to lighting issues, one of which is the ambient noise caused by the fans in lights. He explained that while one used to deal with 72 lighting channels, nowadays the lighting systems and equipment are much more complex and provide stunning lighting possibilities that can require more than 800 channels. The new equipment, however, also poses many technical difficulties in terms of ambient noise.

Lights in the theater used to require gels to give the light a color. Each light had a fixed color and was set during technical rehearsals. Today, designers often employ color rollers, which allow each conventional light to have many different colors available by means of a string of different color gels. These gel strings can be moved gel by gel in front of the light to give the designer greater flexibility. The movement of the gel strings, however, is noisy and the scroller traps a great deal of the heat from the lamp, requiring fans to cool the lamps down so the gel does not burn through. These are also extremely noisy. In some cases, the gel change can occur during a scene change and can be somewhat obscured by the sound cues of the scene change but, in other cases, the light change may be designed to occur during an actual scene on stage and the noise can be extremely distracting. Depending on where the light is hung and whether it is a thrust stage or proscenium, the noise can create quite a distraction. Particularly in a thrust, such as the Festival Theatre at Stratford, the lights are situated in such a fashion that both audience and actors can hear the fans and the noise of the gel strings moving; and in a proscenium stage, such as the Avon Theatre, also at the Stratford Shakespeare Festival, the lights are mostly hung above the stage and therefore primarily distracting to the actors. In both instances, this can be problematic, detracting from the intimacy of the scenes portrayed.

Darker gels cause more heat to get trapped in the lamp and therefore require more fanning; otherwise, the gels will melt, snapping the gel string and potentially creating even more noise. Depending on the quality and age of the scroller, adjustments can be made to mitigate the noise problem. Manufacturers have been aware of the problem from the introduction of the technology and continue to develop quieter fans and the ability to control the fan speed (low, medium, and high, like a hair dryer); they can even be preset to periodically turn the fan off. That way, if a light cue is set for a scene that needs to be quiet, the fan can be turned off for that scene.

Moving lights, which can be controlled by computer to refocus and change color, provide the designer still greater flexibility, but can also create significant noise problems. Many moving lights have a lamp, which burns at a very high temperature and requires four to six fans that need to run all the time. There are moving lights with tungsten bulbs that do not use a fan but are not as bright either, so these lights can be quite annoying if the play involves any nuance or intimacy in terms of content. In addition, the internal motors that control the movement of the fixtures create noise of their own.

Theater companies interested in investing in any kind of technology should consider carefully the balance between budget, enhanced quality of productions, and the needs of actors and audience members before they arrive at the appropriate solution for their venue or a particular production. The most appropriate solution to any situation is likely to involve an approach that utilizes the expertise of theater consultants, acoustics specialists, production managers, and voice specialists. Theater companies need to keep abreast of the most advanced equipment as the market changes year to year. Obviously, artistic directors need to decide if the fancy lights are suited to the kind of work the company produces or not. If they are, producers should work with consultants and specialists in lighting technology and acoustics to research the lighting equipment best suited to their needs. It is best to purchase the most flexible and high-end lighting equipment possible with the greatest degree of noise mitigation features and make sure this is included in the projected budget.

Often, these problems do not emerge until the production is underway. The director and vocal coach do well to research the equipment before the actors move into the theater, so they can troubleshoot any problems that might arise. Ideally, these are issues that need to be addressed when a theater is being designed.

Another issue is the sound caused by equipment used for cooling and heating systems, which can also prove extremely troublesome for theaters that emphasize the clarity of the spoken word. Simon Marsden, Technical Director at the Stratford Shakespeare Festival, informs me that the Festival administration, under the guidance of Antoni Cimolino, General Director of the Festival, has hired various acoustics specialists to assess the acoustics at the Festival. The administration and these specialists are doing comparative studies with other classical companies in the Unites States and United Kingdom. The creative team at the Festival is now working closely with these acoustics specialists on long-range planning to minimize ambient noise caused by electrical equipment or heating and cooling systems. The lighting equipment purchased for the theater can be turned off during scenes to minimize the impact of any electrical noise. The company is dedicated to the spoken word and hearing the spoken word without amplification, in its pure form.

Theatre for a New Audience, under the artistic direction of Jeffrey Horowitz, will soon begin the construction of a new building in Brooklyn, and acoustics specialists have been employed to work with the architects and engineers to minimize the ambient sound in order to honor the purity of the spoken word, again without amplification.

These various acoustical problems do require special attention. My hat goes off to the administrators who take the time and effort to address these issues to create optimum conditions to allow the beauty of language to be spoken in the most acoustically balanced environment as possible. The most sophisticated microphone in the world can never improve on the authentic, vital, and unencumbered sound expressed by an actor in an acoustically live space.

Corsets

When actors (usually female, but sometimes male) wear corsets, the challenge is to maintain proper support. Women used to faint when corsets were commonly worn because the corsets cut off their breath supply. At the fitting, the actor must expand her ribs as fully as possible, keeping them expanded throughout the fitting. There is no need to mention this to the designer or cutter. A good designer knows actors need to feel at ease on stage in the costume. Occasionally, designers and costume people become so focused on the line of the costume that they forget the person inside it actually has to breathe, move, and function on stage like a human being. (As an actress, I was fitted once into a costume so tight, my skin began to bleed around the sleeve seam in the underarms of the costume. I was then able to get the necessary adjustment made.)

A number of years ago at the Stratford Festival, the Alexander staff observed that the actresses wearing corsets were developing a band of tension around their lower ribs. This was brought to the attention of the designers and cutters, who then put more attention into creating the illusion of the desired line for the costume without hindering the actual movement of the ribs.

Carol Miller, one of the senior cutters at the Stratford Shakespeare Festival, explained to me that the main goal of the corset is to achieve the appropriate silhouette historically accurate to the period. She added,

> However, because we are dealing with modern women with modern bodies, used to wearing sweat pants and tee shirts, we

need to always make sure the actor is comfortable. We adjust to each actor as each corset is individually constructed. We often used stretch panels, especially for singers. When we take the measurements, we take the bust and the ribs in full swing so we mold the corset to the shape of the individual. Generally we use flexbone, which is made of metal that spirals so it can move. We often use nylon flexbones for the bodice except in the case of a long bodice that shapes in a triangle to the lower front pelvis. These need to remain flat so we use a steel bone in the center of the bodice to maintain the shape. If the corset is cut properly, the fabric is stretched up and down, and the corset holds the shape of the costume, rather than the costume itself. We take pride in making the corsets adjustable to the comfort of the actor.

Suzy Q. Campbell, Professor of Design at Kent State, designed a corset with a pouch in the front diaphragm, thereby allowing the actor more flexibility in terms of breath support.

When an actor wears a corset, she needs to get in touch with the lower support muscles of the abdomen and back pelvis area. She must keep the belly released as well as the muscles of the pelvis. It helps the integration of breath support and good voice usage if the actors can wear the corsets during rehearsals and at voice tutorials, along with rehearsal skirts and the shoes used in the production. The more the actor can accustom herself to the corset in rehearsal, the more successfully she adapts to any alignment and support challenges. However, it is best to warm up *not* wearing the corset. See Appendix at the end of this chapter for a specific warm-up designed for preparation in a show that involves wearing a corset.

MOUSTACHES

Moustaches can obscure text clarity. The most important thing for the actor, coach, and director to remember is that the actor must articulate aggressively yet without vocal pushing when sporting a moustache; otherwise, the text sounds, particularly consonants, become muffled. He should use enough glue so as not to worry the moustache will fall off. Then he can move his mouth comfortably and as much as needed to enunciate, without distraction to his focus or clarity.

Masks

Usually full masks are only used without dialogue. Using text with half masks can prove challenging because the mask absorbs the resonance around the face, preventing the sound from carrying as effectively. Using the YBuzz and humming in the face help warm up the lower part of the face resonators. The actor can pay particular attention to the head resonator as well, especially the back of the head. If the mask includes a headpiece, then the actor should think of the sound releasing out the back of the neck. The masked actor must pay special attention to articulation, exaggerating it slightly to compensate for the mask's tendency to create a muffled sound.

Child Actors

Several years ago, I coached in a situation where a child had been cast in a fairly substantial role. The child had no acting background. The director told me the child had a "little lisp" but had been able to make a clear *s* at the audition, so the director was confident the child could manage the Shakespearean text. In fact, this child could not make an *s* without enormous jaw tension, as he had a bad overbite. He was also missing his front teeth, which created difficulty for him in speaking the sounds *sh*, *n*, *t*, *d*, *l*, and any other sounds where the tongue needs to be precise in its relationship to the teeth and hard palate. This had a huge impact on his clarity, particularly because he was dealing with Shakespearean text. Many hours were spent in coaching sessions trying to address this speech defect, which normally would require sessions with a speech pathologist, but the theater was not willing to pay for such services. I coached the child but improvement was slow. He also did not have any prior voice training and was attempting to fill a 2,000-seat house, a daunting task even for many experienced actors.

Over the weeks the young boy did improve and become loud enough, as he was quite diligent about practicing the exercises I gave him. However, many sounds related to his speech impediment were still unintelligible. The director suggested a microphone. I explained that using a microphone would only amplify the fact that his diction was poor. The difficulty was text clarity. The microphone also would have resulted in a different sound quality from the rest of the cast. We were able, finally, to get him to an acceptable level of intelligibility, through many hours of coaching, cumulatively many more hours than leads in the show received. Fortunately, this was the sweetest child, who was willing to put in the practice. Nonetheless, the coaching needed to be ongoing throughout the entire 6-month run and the child never quite made it up to a professional level.

When employing child actors, it is extremely helpful to invite the vocal coach to the auditions and elicit his feedback regarding the feasibility of the child successfully meeting the demands of the role. Wherever possible, it is best to begin voice and text coaching before the child begins rehearsals in order to give the child enough time to integrate the work with some confidence. Children generally have to keep up with their schoolwork at the same time, so the coach and director need to be aware that the child will not be available for coaching to the same degree a professional actor is. The child normally does not integrate the work as quickly as an experienced professional, so the theater (or film) needs to allot extra time for coaching sessions. When a child is put into a situation in which he has little chance of success, it is hard on the child's self-esteem and bad for the overall artistic success and morale of the production. The director needs to educate himself about challenges to free voice use and, wherever possible, seek out the help of an experienced and reputable professional coach to assist in making intelligent casting choices and setting realistic goals within the coaching schedule.

I dialect coached a television show where I was responsible for guiding a young 16-year-old actress to master an American dialect for an American show being shot in Canada. This young Canadian woman was working on several television productions while attempting to maintain her studies in school. She did not understand why the producers wanted her to learn the dialect and was resistant to mastering it. She was also exhausted and just wanted to sleep when we were booked to have sessions. The film and television actors associations have guidelines as to how many hours persons under 21 can rehearse and it is extremely important these guidelines are followed so as to avoid this sort of unfortunate situation. She thought the American dialect sounded "stupid" and didn't seem to understand that if the producers wanted her to learn it, that this was part of her job. Finally I convinced her to do it, just so the producers would "leave her alone" and she seemed to appreciate the logic of this idea. Sometimes one is as much a psychologist as a coach. Had the coach been involved at the onset of casting, however, some of these problems could have been avoided. The coach could have briefed the actress as to what to expect during the course of the shooting and work with her on an ongoing basis, rather than having to squeeze in the time between takes, when the actor was over tired.

Summary

Actors tend to respond best to technical challenges when they know about them early in rehearsal and wherever possible have the opportunity to work with these during the rehearsal period. Obviously, that is not possible with fog, but often one can incorporate sound cues, corsets, shoes, wigs, possibly moustaches and heavy costume pieces earlier in the rehearsal process, as these often impact the actor's alignment and, hence, the actor's voice. When I was coaching on a show Martha Henry was directing, the artistic director wanted to cut a costume piece, a cape. I was impressed that Henry's main concern was how this would impact the actor's performance, especially because this request occurred the night before opening. Many directors would not have considered the impact on the actor but, of course, because Henry is such an experienced and brilliant actress herself, she did. Of course, not every director necessarily has to have acted—although it is a huge help—to learn sensitivity to these sorts of issues. Wherever possible, theaters do well to hire a voice and/or Alexander coach for help in dealing with these kinds of challenges.

APPENDIX

Vox Explora or Vocal Preparation for Performing with a Corset

Performing with a corset poses special challenges because of the increased difficulty of finding one's proper breath support with the constriction of the ribs due to the corset.

As stated earlier, nowadays, good designers and cutters pride themselves in making corsets for actors that are specifically tailored to the actor's body. Nonetheless, directors should be aware that the corset challenges the actor vocally and that actors need to adjust the vocal warm-up accordingly.

Here is a warm-up to help actors prepare for performing in a corset. Although primarily women use corsets, men occasionally are costumed in corsets for a particular period or if the actor is playing a "gender bender" role as in *Cloud Nine* by Caryl Churchill.

Warm-Up to Prepare for Performing with a Corset

Start lying on the floor, with the knees bent, feet flat on the floor and the knees directed toward the ceiling.

Imagine that the sacrum is a clock (the sacrum is at the bottom of the spine, just above and including the tailbone) and that the top of the sacrum, nearest the head, is 12 o'clock and the bottom is 6 o'clock.[1] Then the side of the sacrum to the right-hand side is 3 o'clock and to the left-hand side is 9 o'clock. First, rock from 12 to 6, first without sound, just on breath, and then with sound on *huh*, imagining the sound releasing out the sacrum, as if it is pouring into the floor below. Then repeat going from 3 o'clock to 9 o'clock, first on breath and then on sound. Then repeat going from 12 to 6, past 9 in a big half moon, first on breath and then on sound. Then go from 6 to 12, past 9, in a half moon, first on breath, then on sound. Then do a full circle, first on breath and then on sound, first clockwise, then counterclockwise. The sacrum should

---

[1] This is an exercise inspired by Moishe Feldenkrais' work.

feel activated and the sound "dropped." It's important not to force this but to let the sound release easily.

Then go up into the preparation for the bridge, lifting vertebra by vertebra until you are on the shoulders and you clasp your hands stretched out underneath you. Then unclasp one's hands and come down vertebra by vertebra, until the full back is on the floor. Sense the width and length of the back. Notice the movement of the back ribs.

A variation of this is to put a ball (about 6 inches in diameter) under the sacrum, with the knees pointed toward the ceiling. This helps center the breath and release tension in the back. Depending on the comfort level, one can keep the ball under the sacrum for 5 to 10 minutes and then mindfully remove it, placing the back gently on the floor. Usually one finds more sense of length and width in the back, as well as a deeper connection to the breath.

Then lift the pelvis slightly off the ground, thinking of the knees away from you and the feet into the floor. Here is a good place to include some of the Fitzmaurice floor exercises.

Another alternative is to gently sigh out on *huh* and gentle humming, rocking the head from side to side. Imagine the sound of the hum starting at the sacrum and moving up the spine, out the top of the head, thinking of the sound massaging the spine as one goes. Then imagine the sound vibrations of the hum starting in the skull and moving down the spine to the sacrum. Do this a few times and then imagine the sound flowing out of the pelvis area.

One can experiment with different pitches here and then take the hum onto different vowel sounds, making sure to allow a lot of vibration in the lips when they are closed, before one opens them. It's important to keep the release of sound gentle and think of the whole body producing the sound, so as not to push from the tongue root, causing forcing from the throat. Release; go over into the prayer position slowly and mindfully. Touch sound, thinking of the openness of the sacrum. Place hands on the buttocks and feel the subtle expansion of the muscles of the pelvic floor as the breath comes in and the gentle contraction as the breath releases.

One might return again to some of the Fitzmaurice floor exercises here.

Then release the legs, hug the knees to the torso, and roll over gently and mindfully into the prayer position; touch sound.

Then roll over onto your back and hug the knees to the chest. Drop the knees, bent, over to the right on a diagonal stretch, looking toward the other direction. Notice the release in the pelvic muscles and the side ribs. Sigh out on *huh* or *hah* or *hey*. Then reverse this on the other side.

Go onto all fours, bringing the right foot to the right hand, and then the left foot to the left hand, and go into the squat. Make sure the knees are directed over the baby toes so as not to strain the knee joints. Drop the tailbone and sense the pelvic muscles releasing. Then sigh out on *huh*. Bring the sitting bones or ischia (the bones on the bottom of each side of the pelvis on either side of the tailbone) toward the ceiling and drop the torso over, with the neck muscles released. Then uncurl through the spine, head coming up last. Sense the width and ease in the pelvis.

Imagine the sound releasing from the pelvis on an easy sigh on *huh* or *hey*, doing a figure 8 with the hips. Move the sacrum from 6 o'clock to noon as you sigh out on "Hey famousa, kon kon deeky adesa day famousa, kon kon kala," which is a sort of mating call. Really imagine the sound dropping into the pelvis.

Then one can continue stretching the ribs and going on to the resonators and range work as one would normally do, paying extra attention to the width of the pelvis and the lower breath support.

Do the rib stretch as outlined in the Vox Explora in Chapter 5, page 73. Then touch on each resonator gently:

Mouth on *huh*

Chest/back on *hah*

Teeth on *hee*

Ybuzz on *yee-yee-yee*

Sinus on *hee*

Nasal on *mee, may mah*

Head on *kee*

Blow through the lips on *br-br-brumuh*, starting high in pitch and then going as low as you can without pushing down in the larynx. Swing the body, move the hips, keeping this fluid and easy.

You can add text work and gentle speech work here, specific to the performance needs at hand.

The main goal of this warm-up is to make sure the body is loose, especially below the navel, adding awareness of the release of pelvic diaphragm muscles and ease in the legs to adequately compensate for the possible constriction of the ribs caused by the corset. The French call the pelvis *le basin* as in the word *basin*, which is a useful way to think of the pelvis. Spending some extra time to strengthen the connection of the lower breath support helps maintain vocal ease while wearing a corset and gives the actor more vocal confidence.

CHAPTER 10

Working with Voice/Dialect and Alexander Coaches

NEGOTIATION

Voice/Dialect Coaches

A director lucky enough to work with a voice coach should include the coach in the process of rehearsal as much as possible, while at the same time showing sensitivity to the coach's time and salary. Theaters often skimp on voice coach salaries. Directors do well to strongly encourage theater administrators to budget appropriately to pay the vocal coach well. A good rule of thumb for voice coach salary is actor's equity scale and a half or double scale wherever possible. The bare requirement should be at least the equity minimum.

Vocal/dialect coaches (or consultants) should be included in the front page of the program alongside the director, designer, stage manager, and such. In some cases, if the coach has contributed more than 50 hours, it may be appropriate to list her as the voice/dialect/text director (see Preface). If the production involves a big cast and a lot of text and/or dialect work, then use of the term *voice/text* (and possibly *dialect*) *director* reflects most accurately the coach's contribution. Generally, the vocal coach negotiates billing before the production begins, but anything the director can do to underline the importance of the coach to the administration of the theater helps enormously.

When I coached at the Stratford Festival, a wonderfully gifted actress, Joyce Campion, fell off the balcony during a rehearsal of *Macbeth* in the Festival Theatre. She was seriously injured, and for a time there was a question as to whether she would live or die. Fortunately, she recovered. However, her voice was traumatized from the experience and she needed extra vocal work during her recovery period. We worked together for several months after the accident, and it was one of the most gratifying coaching experiences I have ever had. Over time, Ms. Campion not only regained her full vocal strength but found wonderful nuances with increased range and vocal freedom.

At the time, however, it occurred to me that if I had been the unfortunate person to fall off the balcony or somehow injure myself in the theater, there was no compensation in place. I approached the Stratford/Canadian Actors' Equity Liaison committee to see if the voice coaches who were already equity members could be included on an equity contract, and Canadian Actors' Equity (CAE) agreed. Now CAE allows voice coaches to use equity contracts—the same as those used to contract assistant directors. The contract does not specify hours, breaks, or salary but does allow CAE to make contributions toward the coach's retirement plan. The theater also pays a minimal weekly fee while the coach is contracted to provide insurance against injuries. This protects the theater as well as the artist. Subsequent to this, I worked at Canadian Stage for several years as voice and dialect coach for the Shakespeare productions in the park and in each instance I was hired on an equity contract, providing insurance in case of an injury on theater premises. This could save the administration from a messy legal situation if there ever was an accident.

For film and television contracts in Canada, the Association of Canadian Television and Radio Artists (ACTRA) allows ACTRA contracts for coaches who are ACTRA members. ACTRA contracts for coaches use the same scale and a half as singers are contracted for as the basic minimum daily rate. The coach is certainly entitled to negotiate above and beyond this rate, as the market will bear. The contract then covers insurance and retirement contributions. Screen Actors Guild (SAG), Actors' Equity, and American Federation of Television and Radio Artists (AFTRA) hopefully may provide the same opportunity for coaches in the United States, but to date have not done so. Members of the Voice and Speech Trainers Association (VASTA), including Phil Thompson (President of VASTA), Dudley Knight, and I have investigated this possibility. Many directors frequently end up as artistic or associate artistic directors, and therefore are well advised to familiarize themselves with such contractual information, and support vocal coaches in order that coaches receive appropriate benefits and insurance protection wherever possible.

TIPS FOR THE DIRECTOR AND THE VOICE/DIALECT COACH

Prerehearsal Meetings

Assuming that the theater in question pays the coach appropriately, the director and the coach should meet to discuss voice and dialect goals before rehearsals begin. If the director is directing for a repertory company, it is a professional courtesy to contact the resident voice coach as early as possible before rehearsals begin, so the coach can plan accordingly. The resident vocal coach or head of voice in a repertory situation often needs to juggle vocal/dialect requirements for a number of productions and voice training programs for apprentice actors and, in some situations, working with understudies. Highly experienced actors require vocal support as well, including voice tutorials, text consultations, and vocal warm-ups. The resident coach often supervises other coaches, which includes assessing which coach's talents are most appropriate for specific productions and working with particular productions; thus, any information the director can provide regarding the vocal needs of a production ahead of time is of enormous help for the resident coach. If the production requires dialect work, there are child actors in the show, or there are any outstanding vocal demands for the actors, such as a high-intensity scene, fight choreography that might require fight sounds, and so on, this is all useful for the resident coach or assigned coach on the production to know ahead of time.

If possible, in a repertory situation the coach assigned to the show and the director should establish a dialogue before rehearsals. This dialogue is especially important in any show using microphones and/or numerous sound effects. In the case of musicals, it is in the director's best interest to encourage communication among the sound designer, sound technicians, the musical director, and the vocal coach. The vocal coach is an important component to the team and can help enormously to ensure clarity in the spoken dialogue and in the lyrics of the songs, especially those dealing with plot points. The director can encourage this by asking for and taking seriously the coach's input during group discussions. The coach can play an important role in maintaining clarity of text and the acoustic balance of elements like sound effects and orchestras. The director does well to reinforce this.

Once Rehearsals Start

The director should introduce the voice coach on the first day of rehearsal. The director should explain to the cast how important the voice work is and how important it is that they take advantage of the voice person's input. The director can ask for the coach's input during the rehearsal discussion. The director should, ideally, meet with the coach on a weekly basis, even if only for 15 to 30 minutes, to make sure things are on track and that the director and coach are on the same page. If the director does not know to do this, the coach needs to be assertive and make the request while being sensitive that the director has to juggle many other concerns in the production. Remember, the more connected the voices, the better the production. The better the production, the more recognition the director gets. So, any support the director gives the coach ultimately reflects positively on the director.

If the show requires dialects or accents, then the coach usually gives the actors materials on the dialect or accent involving specific sound changes and specific inflection and rhythm changes related to each dialect or accent. If all the cast members are doing the same dialect or accent, the coach may wish to schedule group sessions to go over the basic principles of each one, or, if it involves many different dialects or accents, she may just go straight into one-on-one tutorials to work in detail with each actor.

If the coach can be at the first reading, it helps reinforce her contribution to the show. The cast should never feel as if the coach is a stranger in the rehearsal hall. I spoke with an actor who complained bitterly of a coach who had not been to any rehearsals until the first preview, and gave the actors a great many notes on the dialect. The actors felt thrown off, found it difficult to incorporate the notes, and in some cases perceived the notes as being in conflict with what the director had requested of the actors. The perception was that this total stranger who had not had prior input into the show suddenly appeared to critique it, and, rather than helping the actors master the demands of the dialect with more confidence, merely managed to get the actors rattled. At this point, a coach can cause more harm than good.

Every coach rehearses a little differently. In my experience, the coach can benefit from hearing the first reading in order to troubleshoot potential problems that will then be discussed with the director. However, the coach should bear in mind that the director may feel a little protective and defensive about the casting choices, so it is best for the coach to begin by stating a few positive observations that are truthful before one jumps into any that are critical. The coach should bear in mind as well that a great deal occurs between first reading and opening and closing nights. Many actors shine at the first reading and then never go beyond that level. Others can seem lost for a couple of weeks and then pull everything together to create a beautiful performance. I once heard an interview with Hume Cronyn, who described the process for the late Jessica Tandy. He prided himself on incorporating props and other "business" early, while she would often have her head buried in her script and seem quite muddled. Then she would miraculously one day appear in rehearsal with a spectacular and detailed performance. Thus, it is important not to judge too quickly. Each actor rehearses differently, and sometimes the same actor has quite a different process from production to production, as there are so many variable factors.

The coach generally sits in on rehearsals in order to understand the director's vision and reinforce what the director is striving for. However, a coach is not usually needed during blocking rehearsals, unless a lot of text interpretation occurs.

One-on-One Tutorials

The most productive time to meet with the actors for tutorials is the period from when the show is blocked and the actors are solidly off book until technical rehearsals. If the show involves dialects, then the coach and actor might well meet at the onset of rehearsals, or earlier, so the coach can guide the actor in the basic dialect/accent change, give examples of native speakers, etc. At this time, the actors and director tend to still be exploring, so the coach's input is really valuable. (Also see Chapter 8, Voice and Text Explorations.)

Generally, coaches work with the actors one-on-one in tutorials. Individual sessions should run no less than 30 minutes, ideally 40, unless the coach requests otherwise. These should be included in the official calls and schedules, like fittings and fight calls, on the call sheet. Directors and stage management need to make clear that voice sessions are part of rehearsal. Actors should contact the stage management regarding tutorial time or any changes. This is generally more professional than if the actor contacts the coach directly, unless there is some particular emergency or other specific reason to do so.

It is important that director and stage manager respect that tutorial time. I have often arranged a coaching session, at the request of the director, only to have it interrupted after 10 minutes. Of course, sometimes this simply can't be helped, but where possible directors and stage management should avoid interrupting or short-changing tutorials, as it undermines the work of the coach. A coach cannot work by osmosis. There is no point in a director complaining about an actor's vocal issue if the director is not willing to give the coach time to work with the person.

The tutorials should, ideally, occur in a quiet space with a mat, with enough room for floor work and a piano. I say ideally because, unfortunately, one has to make do with less than ideal conditions to work in. Before the Stratford Festival was renovated I coached in the tiny storeroom for the beverages off the lobby. We would need to turn off the refrigerator to work. This kind of extreme compromise is not recommended. I believe it was not until the late William Hutt complained about his tutorial in the beverage room that the members of the higher administration realized they should make a change! Now the Stratford Shakespeare Festival has improved tutorial spaces considerably, much to the advantage of the acting company and directors. One wants to make available the best spaces possible, in order that the coach can provide the best guidance to the actors.

At one point as a coach working in New York, where of course space is at a great premium, I was giving the leading actor his vocal warm-up in the hallway, where other actors were chatting at the coffee machine. This was extremely distracting. When the actor wanted Alexander classes in the theater, we had great difficulty finding appropriate space. We tried working in a hallway off the dressing rooms and then were told we could not because of fire regulations; we finally ended up working in an aisle behind the audience in the changeover between the two shows. This was an actor who is famous and has won numerous honors in his career and we still could not find proper space to work in! Of course, one does one's best whatever the space issue, but wherever possible, the theater should provide an appropriate space to coach, even if this involves a budget increase. Any support from the director to get better spaces for tutorials is of great help to the productions.

In the one-on-one tutorial, time can be devoted to voice work that involves taking the actor through a series of vocal exercises, depending on what her vocal needs are. (Many of the explorations are listed in chapters 5, 6, and 7.) If a dialect or accent is required, normally one reviews the basic changes involved with the actor and then goes through the text, guiding her in applying these changes. It is best to integrate the dialect or accent work with a lot of text work, so that the dialect or accent becomes seamlessly integrated with the acting. It is great when the director and coach are working closely, hand in glove.

For example, it can take the actor a couple of rehearsals to integrate the work in the tutorial. The director needs to understand that the voice and text work is not an overnight process, so if the director has asked the voice coach to work on a specific area, the work of the tutorial may not appear to take hold immediately. As mentioned earlier, some aspects of the work may cause an actor to slow down for a short time, so it is helpful if the director can give a little latitude in this regard. This benefits both the actor and the show.

If no dialect is required, then one can devote time to text work. In *The Merchant of Venice* and *The Jew of Malta*, produced by Theatre for a New Audience, we had the luxury of an extended rehearsal period, so I was able to go through the bulk of the text with most of the actors. We explored the imagery and its visceral connection to the text, the iambic pentameter, support issues, getting the build of the thoughts clear, articulation, and getting the sound rooted and forward in the mask. This is a time when it is valuable for the coach and director to touch base so they can reinforce each other's work—and for the coach to sit in on pertinent rehearsals.

The point is that it is important, as much as possible, for everyone to be on the same page. As a coach, it is fine to summarize and hit the high points for the director. Most directors have a lot on their plates and the support a coach offers benefits the acting ensemble and the director.

Time

As stated earlier, the most useful time for the coach's contribution occurs once the show is blocked and the actors are off book, but still exploring. Sometimes directors bring coaches into the process when it is too late for the actor to successfully make any adjustments. It is important that the coach's contributions are synchronized with the time period when the actors are solidly off book and working in depth but things are not too set. Of course, a good coach is sensitive to time and can make a positive contribution at any point in rehearsal, but this is really an optimum period to have a helpful impact. Again, the director needs to give the coach adequate time with the actor. There is no point in a director saying, "So-and-so has a terrible diction problem," and then not give the coach adequate time to address the problem.

Notes

A voice coach does not usually give notes on individual scenes, unless an actor or director specifically requests the coach to do so or there is some particular vocal issue, such as the actor needs to scream or tends to push vocally. One does take notes on run-throughs of acts and full run-throughs of the play, assuming the director schedules these in. Usually, one does not take notes on the first run-through unless it is the only one scheduled before technical rehearsals. The ideal is to take notes on the second run-through, so the actors have had a chance to incorporate blocking, use of props, and so on. If run-throughs are scheduled back to back for several days, generally the coach should take notes on every second or third run-through so as to give the actors an opportunity to integrate the notes, without the sense that the coach is breathing down their necks.

The notes consist of letting the actor know what is working vocally, that is, feedback such as, "This is a good vocal level" and "This section is clear." With a big cast, it is not always possible to "catch the actor doing something right" as often as one would like, simply because one does not have enough hands to write everything quickly enough. In these instances, one lets the actors know the lines and, in some cases, the words that are not clear. It's helpful to follow along with the script and give the page number and, if possible, the line number, so the actor can go back and check it. These details help the actors know exactly where and what they need to focus on. If the actor is dealing with a dialect or accent, then it is appropriate to give her specific notes on the sounds and inflections. If the actor knows the International Phonetic Alphabet symbols, then it is fine to use those. If the actor is not familiar with these, then dictionary symbols or indicating a sound with a commonly used word or regular spelling works. For example, if one wants the actor to make the "a" sound as in the word *cat*, it helps to give the actor the specific sound. This becomes more difficult with sounds that North Americans do not use, such as the British *ah* sound in *ask*. This is where CDs of native speakers can aid actors in learning the appropriate sounds for specific dialects, and then the dialect coach can refer the actor to the relevant sections of the CDs. When the actor comes to the next tutorial, one can utilize the time to review the notes and guide the actor in fine-tuning her performance.

A coach should take notes during runs of the play in the rehearsal hall as technical rehearsals are approaching. At this point, actors can integrate the notes because they generally have not become too set in their interpretation. If the text is clear in the rehearsal hall, generally the actor can make the adjustment to a larger house without too much difficulty. If the text is not clear in the final rehearsal, or it is vocally pushed, one can usually assume that the lack of text clarity and pushing will remain or worsen in the theater. Thus, it is important these issues are addressed as much as possible before the move into the theater. The director and stage manager should remind the actors to review the voice coach's notes, particularly during tech week. Sometimes the coach may give general notes after the director's notes, such as, "Make sure to use the final words of the thoughts and the final consonants of the final words" or "We are losing some of the clarity on stage left because of the pillar," but specific, individual notes are best written up for each actor so the actor can refer back to these notes at a later date. The coach should hear what the director's notes are, so that these can be reinforced and understood in giving the voice or dialect notes. The coach can write these up on recipe cards, or 3" × 5" note cards.[1]

There is little point in the coach giving notes during technical rehearsals except if the show has a great many sound cues that might obscure the clarity of the text. These notes are best given to the director, rather than the actors. The other instance when the coach might need to take notes during technical rehearsals would be if the show were microphoned and/or the production is a musical in which one must balance speaking with the clarity of song lyrics. In these situations, the coach can offer valuable feedback to the director, musical director, sound director, and technicians. The voice coach may give notes that relate to sound or music levels to the director and/or the musical director during technical rehearsals and previews. Once the show has opened, these notes should be given to the stage manager. If, however, the sound designer, sound technician(s), and coach have established a positive rapport, then it may be fine for the coach to give the notes directly to them and, as a professional courtesy, copy the notes to the stage manager. This latter situation generally proves best for the overall sound and vocal quality of the production, but involves a judgment call on the part of the coach. It is usually best to err on the side of diplomacy unless one is certain.

Coaching the dialects and lyrics for *Boyfriend* at the Stratford Festival, I was fortunate that the sound technicians sought out the expertise of the vocal coach, which was of great benefit to the show. In addition, musical director Bert Carrière and director Brian Macdonald were supportive of the voice coach's contributions, which also helped the actors enormously.

Usually, the coach can return to give notes after the second dress rehearsal. Actors tend to get understandably distracted by their costumes at the first dress, so this is usually not the best time to give notes unless one has absolutely no other opportunity. Giving notes in previews is tricky. At that point, it is best to really think

---

[1] A great idea given to me by Mary Hartley, Pittsburgh, PA.

carefully about the importance of each note in terms of the actor's overall performance. Framing notes in a manner that reinforces what works well and encouraging the actor to go further is the best approach at this point, but without being so specific that the actor becomes self-conscious about particular sections. In fact, sometimes extremely specific notes, good or bad, can undermine an actor's performance, rendering the actor self-conscious. Notes at this point should have to do with dead spots in the house. One might miss an end of a line or chunks of lines. There does come a point where the actor has to play the scene, and too much meddling can get in the way of the actor's process. On the other hand, it is the actor's responsibility to be heard and understood. Coaches cannot be too concerned with popularity contests, as it is not unusual for actors to get prickly near opening night. Giving notes by e-mail is not a bad idea, so the actor can choose when she reads them, and this allows the coach a bit of distance. Notes throw some actors more easily than others, so the coach needs to make a judgment call. (And to any actors reading this: coaches are human and make mistakes too, so cut them the same slack before an opening that they do for you.) Directors should be aware of this in terms of their notes as well. Most actors integrate notes after tech with minimal success. In most cases, directors and coaches do well to back off during previews, unless some serious problem needs to be addressed.

Usually, musical theater performers are extremely comfortable with notes at any juncture. In fact, at Stratford, I found the musical theater performers got a little edgy if you did *not* have notes for them! As the production goes into previews, the good coach gives encouraging notes, rather than notes that are too "corrective." A good rule of thumb for coaches: give the notes no more than three times. Sometimes an actor simply is not capable of something. Perhaps she forgets, or she simply doesn't have the technical ability. As the show progresses, it is necessary for the coach (and the director) to practice sensitivity in terms of the relative importance of a specific note compared to the overall confidence of the actor. The actor finally has to play the scene, not the note.

The main point here is that the more involved the voice coach is, the more she can tune in to the frame of mind of the cast and contribute to the overall success of the show; thus, it behooves the director and other artists involved with the production to take advantage of the voice coach's expertise. The coach has to determine on a case-by-case basis how to best contribute, being aware that in the theater one always has to be careful of the various egos and territorial concerns. One can put a foot wrong unintentionally quite easily and ruffle someone's feathers without meaning to. One then has to determine whether it is important to address the situation directly or just move on as quickly as possible. There is no perfect answer, so this is where the coach's sensitivity comes into play.

BOUNDARIES

It is important that the director support the contributions of the vocal coach both in the rehearsal hall and in any social situations as well.

It is also important to mention that on occasion coaches are overly judgmental, or have forgotten or have perhaps never experienced the difficulties of acting or directing. Some voice and dialect coaches work in a rather "shame-based" manner. This means that they overemphasize a right/wrong attitude, intimating, "Why don't you have this yet?" The actor can experience this attitude as undermining and, naturally, this can foster a rather defensive reaction among actors. Actors will then shut off to anything the voice coach says, which is not helpful to the overall production. Voice/dialect coaches need to understand how vulnerable actors are and demonstrate sensitivity in how to approach them and when. Once actors realize a coach is supporting them, my experience is that they will welcome the coach's feedback and ask for particular feedback for trouble spots.

A movement coach I worked with once said, "The amateur coach tells you what is wrong; the professional coach gives you something constructive to do to address it." Most individuals work better within a positive atmosphere. That is not to say one doesn't make demands on actors, but one can do this in a respectful and positive manner. I learned a lot from working with Ted Pappas, Artistic Director of Pittsburgh Public Theater, when I coached *Medea*, starring Lisa Harrow. He was extremely firm when something wasn't working, and insisted the actors address the problem and worked with them until they did, accepting nothing less. When they did master something, he would shower them with praise. This is a good approach. The idea is "The such and such is not yet working" rather than "You are a worthless actor and human being for not getting this yet."

An actor once told me he had had a vocal coach give him a note after the first reading about the optimal pitch of his voice because the coach did not think the actor was speaking at the appropriate pitch. This is a rather old-fashioned idea to begin with, as each person has a range of about three or more octaves, so one should not limit the voice or the thinking about a character in this manner. Perhaps, in all fairness, the coach meant that the actor needed to support the pitch choice more. In any case, a first reading is far too early to give that sort of specific suggestion.

Another actor I worked with, who graduated from a prestigious program in New York, was incredibly defensive. Eventually, I discovered that this was partly because his voice teacher had bullied him in acting school. Alan Rickman, in an interview on NPR's *Fresh Air*, said his voice teacher told him his voice sounded like the back of a drain pipe! Given this kind of teaching and coaching, it is no wonder some actors respond to coaches in a defensive manner and don't wish to work with them.

Sometimes the voice work can cause an actor to become vulnerable in a tutorial. In such a case, the coach does best to respond like a "good friend" just by listening and offering support, something I learned from the gifted Alexander and acting coach Michael Frederick that he learned in his training with the late Walter Carrington. Although the voice is definitely related to the overall psychological aspects of the actor, the coach is not a therapist and should not set herself up as one.

It is important for coaches to respect actors' confidentiality. When working at a reputable repertory company, I was shocked at the way the coaches spoke about the actors, infantilizing them and delving into their personal lives. It is certainly reasonable in a coaching situation to say to another coach something like, "Well, so-and-so is experiencing difficulties in such-and-such at rehearsal, and so you might want to reassure him." But it is inappropriate to discuss details unrelated to the actor's performance, such as whom the actor is involved with or whether or not the actor is having financial or marital problems. It is really none of the coach's business. The actor is always in a vulnerable position professionally—even a successful star—because often the weight of the project rests more on the star's shoulders. Anything said about the actor, even in casual conversation, can be misconstrued and therefore can cause damage. Coaches need to think about the ethics of these situations carefully (as should directors, stage management, production, administrative staff, and actors.[2])

A coach should avoid contradicting a director, not because the director might not be wrong but because this only serves to confuse the actor. When I was playing Titania in a production of *A Midsummer Night's Dream*, I went into a voice tutorial just 2 days before the opening. The coach said to me, "That wig looks awful. And the way he has you blocked—you are being totally upstaged. The scene doesn't work at all." It completely undermined my confidence and was clearly inappropriate on the coach's part. If the coach has strong views about how the production is going or suggestions about staging or costumes, it is best to keep quiet about these unless one has the courage to discuss it with the director. I am embarrassed to say I froze and did not say anything to the coach about how upset I was. Sometimes actors are vulnerable or nervous enough that they may not speak up when something disturbs them. This provides yet another reason for the coach to exhibit an approachable and encouraging manner in rehearsal. The only good news about this aforementioned situation was that afterwards I thought to myself, "Don't ever do that to an actor." And I haven't.

Often in repertory situations, there are a number of coaches. Under these circumstances, it generally works best if one coach is assigned to one show. When more than one coach is working on a show, it can confuse the actors. If more than one coach is unavoidable, because of scheduling or whatever, it is important that the various coaches keep abreast of the notes being given so as not to overload the actors at a given time.

Coaches—especially ones who have never acted—need to realize that actors require time to process suggestions. They need time to focus on one area at time, and can't be expected to integrate everything at once. Once I was in a coaching situation with another

---

[2] I highly recommend the book *The Ethics of Touch* by Ben E. Benjamin and Cherie Sohnen-Moe (published 2005 by Sohnen-Moe Associates). It is written specifically for massage therapists and other body workers, but brings up excellent boundary issues that prove extremely useful for both voice/dialect coaches and Alexander coaches.

VOICE/DIALECT AND ALEXANDER COACHES 179

voice/speech coach and a movement coach. The movement coach was working with the actors and it was the actors' first time in the theater. The other voice/speech coach became concerned that the actors were not breathing, and told the movement coach, which was fine. He continued, however, to tell the movement coach several times and then told the actors several times. I could not help thinking that if the actors had been left to their own devices they might well have begun to breathe more easily on their own, and the constant reminders only served to get them more nervous. Like directors, coaches can become nervous and worry that the actors are not "getting the notes" quickly enough, and sometimes this manifests as over-coaching. It is always good to give some time between notes for the individual to incorporate them. It is easy as a coach to forget how difficult it is for the actor to integrate all the aspects of voice or dialect details into the overall performance. Once an actor realizes the coach is there to help her give the best possible performance, and the coach communicates this support, actors tend to pick this up and relax and then begin asking for feedback, from a trusted ear.

Sometimes actors will try to lure the coach into discussing other actors' performances or other aspects of the production. As a coach, it's best to avoid these discussions. I worked with a coach who constantly spent coaching sessions criticizing the director, who was also the artistic director. She would often talk to me in the halls about it and I was extremely uncomfortable and kept changing the subject. I really did not want to be overheard and perceived as being complicit in this sort of behavior. In retrospect, I should have been more specific in my discomfort, but I reported to this individual and was concerned about the impact it might have on other areas of my work.

Sometimes coaches criticize the directors to the actors. Of course, we are all human and a little of this is understandable. That said, coaches should realize that part of their job is to support the directors as well as the actors. If a coach feels strongly that something needs to be addressed, it is best to pick an appropriate time to bring this up to the director rather than talk about it behind the director's back to the actors or to the other coaches. I once worked in a situation where the coaches complained that the director was not giving enough positive feedback to some of the actors, but seemed quite shocked when I suggested that they might speak to the director face-to-face at an opportune moment. One actor, for example, expressed to me how undermined he felt in rehearsals. He felt the director and one of the stars would discuss the scene without acknowledging his presence, let alone ask for his input. The actor was the only African American in the company and already felt pretty disenfranchised. I saw the director at the cafeteria line and took a deep breath. "Did you notice how John has improved in his voice and text work?" The director said, "Oh, yes." Pause. "Well, I have been working with him . . . " "Oh, great. Thanks." I added, "It would be great if you mentioned to him that you have noticed his improvement." The director stared at me in shock. I went on, "I mean, of course, I have told him, but it means so much more coming from the director." This director has huge brown eyes and stared at me for about 30 seconds but what felt like an eternity. "All right," he finally said. And he did. Once directors get over the initial shock that a vocal coach might actually have something useful to contribute to the process, they often come to depend on these contributions and may even seek them out!

Generally, it is best if a coach does not contradict a director to the actor, as it only serves to confuse the actor and can have a detrimental impact on the production. What the coach can do, however, is understand what the director wants and help an actor find a way to achieve that while honoring healthy voice principles and the actor's integrity. I have made one exception to the rule of not contradicting the director. I was coaching an outdoor Shakespeare production, and we were at the final preview at the end of a long week of technical rehearsals, having spent several days in extremely humid, hot weather. I was sitting in on the note session, and the director told two of the actors that they sounded "odd" and then looked at me and asked, "Don't you agree?" I honestly had no idea what he was talking about and I am quite certain I would have noticed if something had been off.[3] The only thing I heard that night were tired voices from being out in the sun for 12 hours, but no more so with these two actors than any other. One of the actors caught me in the parking lot and the other called me at home late that night.

---

[3] I have a talent and a curse: my ears are so highly sensitive, I hear the show for the first time every time and I can pick up the slightest nuance of a voice disconnected to the thought or the slightest vocal pushing. In fact, one of my former students, the talented actor Danny Bernardy, referred to me as a "polygraph—the slightest insincerity and her ear catches it."

Both were panicked about what the director said. I took a second to think and then I broke my rule of never contradicting the director. I said, "Don't worry about it. You sound fine. Just get some rest. He's just tired." Once in a while, you have to make a judgment call about what is best for the overall show, which in the end is going to help the director!

Ideally, the coach can provide a safe haven to allow the actor to explore vocally and textually, without fear of repercussions, such as losing one's job or not being rehired by a particular theater. The coach serves as an accurate ear that can discern both clarity of thought and proper breath support. Of course, the actor needs to respect the coach's time by showing up promptly and well prepared for tutorials. I usually ask an actor if there is something she would like to work on, and it is gratifying when the actor has given some prior thought to the session and has some specific goals.

Directors' Nerves before Openings

At a repertory company I coached at for a few seasons, there were several shows and the previews were several weeks. Often, the directors would back off the shows at this time. As a coach, one would guide the actors in the text work and help them to find the proper breath support and coach the understudies, and finally, by about a week before opening, the shows were in solid shape and the actors ready to fly into the run with confidence and ease. Then a few days before the official openings, the directors would reemerge and start calling the actors for rehearsals and "reworking things." This included changing staging, cutting lines, adding props, changing sound cues, changing costume pieces and wigs, and even text interpretations. Suddenly the actors, who had begun to gain confidence, became a bundle of nerves, were overly tired, and began to vocally push and become just tense overall, which of course did not help their performances. A director might do well to question whether she really needs to keep tweaking the show up to the last second and risk undermining the actor's overall confidence and, hence, ease in performance. Unfortunately, as the vocal coach, one has to just continue to support and encourage the actors as best as one can, even when the director may be over-meddling with the production. As Tony Soprano would say, "Whadda ya gonna do?"

Group Work

Coaching alongside Cicely Berry on *The Jew of Malta* and *The Merchant of Venice* was an extraordinary experience, and I learned a great deal from the way she worked as well.

She sat by the director and observed a scene. Then there would be a pause and she usually grinned and made a simple but extremely insightful comment such as, "It's about religion here, isn't it?" She would chat a bit to the actors and director and listen carefully to what they said. Then she would devise a "diversion" strategy, as she calls it, fitting for that particular scene. In *The Jew of Malta*, for example, in Act v, scene 2, Barabas (F. Murray Abraham) and Ferneze (Marc Vietor) meet, and Barabas wants to strike a deal with Ferneze. Berry asked two other actors, Kenajuan Bentley and Vince Nappo, to play soldiers guarding Barabas and Ferneze. She instructed one to walk upstage and downstage in the rehearsal hall to stage right of Barabas and Ferneze, and the other to walk downstage and upstage on the stage left side of them. She then instructed the actors that each time one of the guards got near them, they had to lower their voices so the guards could not hear them speak. This had quite an impressive effect. The text became much more specific, and the scene became filled with mystery and danger. By adding this obstacle, the information being communicated became much more important.

I was interested in how Berry worked with the actors as a group, as I tend not to do that a great deal when I coach except in the group warm-ups; I tend to focus more on the one-on-one tutorials, particularly when it is a professional show. Berry's method is a good one and should be employed more often. As the coach's role becomes recognized as more integral to the overall production, I expect coaches can contribute more fully in group work throughout the production process as appropriate.

The next show I coached was with the talented director Mladen Kiselov; I spoke to him about how Berry worked, and we explored this approach quite successfully. Of course, the success of this depends on the situation, and Ms. Berry has the advantage of being one of the most highly respected voice coaches in the world and a great inspirational example.

The main point here is that the more integral to the process the coach is, the more the show benefits from her expertise. Coaches, actors, and directors should think outside the box and look for creative ways to maximize the impact of the voice coach's contribution to the benefit of the whole production.

Communication

The director and coach need to touch base regularly. The coach and actor may spend a session concentrating on breath support, for example. This may result in the actor playing a little more slowly than usual, but it helps if the director can bear with this for a day or so, rather than immediately giving a note requesting a faster pace. The coach obviously needs to let the director know this.

It is important that a director is realistic about what a coach can or cannot do. A coach can help an already well-trained actor achieve a clear, supported performance and assist in issues in articulation as it relates to detailed text work. In a rehearsal of 4 weeks, a coach cannot fix major speech impediments, severe vocal pushing, or an overall lack of technique. However, she can—hopefully—help get the play more clear. She should help the actors attain healthy breath support and clear tone, along with clarity of the text. Sometimes, sadly, one has to resign oneself to simply getting the text as clear as possible. Some actors are so fixed in their ineffective habits that they cannot make appropriate adjustments. As the actor clarifies her thought process, however, often the breath support and vocal tone will improve. My former teacher and colleague David Smukler referred to this as "Band-Aiding."

The process benefits if the director supports the voice work verbally to the actors. For example, when the director gives notes, if something is voice related, add, " . . . as I am sure so-and-so [coach's name] has told you." The better the voices, the better the overall production and the better the director looks. The more the director supports the coach's work, the better the voice in the show. Several years ago, I coached a production of Chekhov's *Three Sisters*, directed by Mladen Kiselov. He spoke about the voice work and my understanding of Chekhov with incredible respect, indeed, almost awe! I felt wonderful, of course, but it also underscored the importance of voice work to the cast, making his, my, and their tasks easier.

I have sometimes worked with directors who overprotect the actors by asking such questions as "Are you okay with voice notes?" or "Are you okay with tutorials?" Yet it would never occur to them to ask an actor, "Are you okay with a fitting today?" or "Do you mind if we start technical rehearsals next week?" Although it is important to show sensitivity to actors, there is no need to indulge them to quite this extent as this undermines the importance of the voice coach's contribution. In one show I coached, the director was terrified to have me give the actors notes because she thought that notes would rattle them. Because I had worked with several of the actors before, they began requesting notes from me, and I had to explain the director didn't want me to give them. Eventually I was able to convince the director that the notes would be valuable to the actors. Ironically, his notes really were upsetting the actors while mine, in fact, were not. I did have a moment of satisfaction when one of the actors thanked me in front of the whole cast and director for the notes and said how helpful they were. This particular actor had told the director that he, the actor, had been frustrated by voice classes in drama school and this was partly why the director was concerned about my working him. This actor, however, had told me the same story at his tutorial and expressed a keen interest in the work we were doing. By over-protecting the actor in this manner, the director was really depriving the actor of a chance to grow in his vocal work. In fact, this actor had a number of vocal issues that he did need help with. The director should trust the coach to do her job and appreciate that a good coach will know to give notes in a sensitive manner, at the appropriate time.

In the same way that coaches should support the director's work, directors should support the coach's work. I worked with Vladimir Mirodan when he directed Chekhov's *Three Sisters*, and he made it perfectly clear on the first day of rehearsal that the actors would be called for voice tutorials and this was the way it was, end of story, and this helped the cast. Of course, Mirodan has the advantage of being married to a brilliant voice and dialect coach, Barbara Berkery.

Some directors like regular communication; some just want the coach to do the work and trust that it gets done. The late Richard

Monette for example, was of the latter category. Generally, it is a good idea for the coach to summarize what she has been working on either by paper or e-mail so the director can refer to it if she chooses to. The coach can gauge how much detail to go into, depending on the director's personality. Usually it is best to hit the high points only and keep it in vocal terms, as some directors get a bit nervous about text work. The coach should, of course, when appropriate, attend the actual rehearsals to observe how the work of the director and the coaching sessions are dovetailing. When coaching *The Jew of Malta* and *The Merchant of Venice* for Theatre for a New Audience, I touched base with the directors quite regularly, either in person or by sending summaries of the work I was doing with the actors by e-mail. When Cicely Berry was working with the company for 2 weeks during November 2006 in New York City during the beginning of *Merchant* rehearsals and toward the end of *Malta* rehearsals, we would speak daily about the work we had done. Because I was with both shows for the full 14 weeks in New York City, from October 30, 2006, to February 11, 2007, naturally I would communicate with Berry on a regular basis by e-mail and phone to keep her abreast of what we were doing. When *Merchant* moved to England after it ran in New York City to sold-out houses, she picked up her work with the cast, doing incredible work with them.

A director needs to listen to the coach's vocal suggestions. I coached *A Midsummer Night's Dream* a number of years ago. The director, also an actor, asked the actors to perform vocally unhealthy tasks. She then became frustrated with the actors when they were unable to achieve what she wanted. She would not listen to any suggestions and then became angry when several of the actors started losing their voices! When this director works as an actor, she generally loses her voice at some point during every run. The person who suffers from voice difficulties often denies it, much like many other problems in life such as alcoholism and drug addiction.

I once coached a show that involved a well-established actor who was quite a challenge. The director and artistic director were pulling their hair out and, to an extent, so was I. The actor had made a point of telling me she reviewed and studied all my notes. I didn't pay much heed until I found out from the artistic director that the director had tried to meet with this actor for 2 weeks to give her notes and the actor refused to meet with the director. The artistic director told me I should not be taking time for tutorials with the actor because the artistic director wanted the actor to devote that time to learning her lines. I had a strong sense that some voice and text work would only help her learn her lines, as in some sections she did not have a full handle on the text. I suggested this and the artistic director made it clear that he thought this work should come from the director. The director had many visual talents; however, he was not strong with text, but I did not feel I could say this to the artistic director. It became a moot point because the actor cancelled the tutorial with me. I had assured the director the actor had a killer instinct and I had no doubt she would be fine by opening week. Time went by and I waited for the director to give these supposed text notes the artistic director told me about, but the director never did, or if he did, it did not materialize on stage. The show went into technical rehearsals, and by previews the actor was blanking on the same lines over and over again.

Unfortunately, the place she was blanking on was in her opening monologue, which shook her confidence at the top of the show. I finally took matters into my own hands and sent her some specific voice and text suggestions about the first monologue by e-mail. In retrospect, perhaps I should have done this sooner or checked with the director, but on the other hand, by waiting the actor may have been in a more receptive state to take them. And by checking with the director, the issues might have become muddy and the solution put off another week or two, by which time it would have been too late. In any case, the actor never acknowledged the notes, but it was obvious from her performance that she had taken the specific suggestions, and the next night her first monologue took off with no memory lapses and set up the rest of her performance beautifully. And yes, even before opening week, the leading actor's killer instinct was well in place and the performance was spectacular.

The Alexander Coach

Many theaters cannot afford Alexander coaches, but for those theaters that can they are a huge asset to a production. The coach gives one-on-one tutorials, and sometimes leads group classes and warm-ups. The coach may attend rehearsals and give notes on alignment issues that crop up in rehearsal. In some situations, the coach can actually participate in the rehearsal and work with actors doing hands-on work with them as they are playing the scene, helping them to find more ease and release. This helps actors to integrate the principles of the Alexander Technique (AT) into their performance in a practical way. This is something the director, coach, and actors would all have to collaborate on and requires a solid trust among all parties. This way of working would be less advisable during runs of acts or run-throughs of the whole show, as it might be too many things to focus on at once for the actor. Again, as the show gets closer to opening, it is more difficult for actors to take in new information. So there is a time for hands on and a time for hands off!

The Alexander coach is available to help actors deal with tension issues that crop up in fight choreography or dance choreography. Good Alexander coaches who work in theater usually have some background in voice and acting, and if the coach does not, she should at least take some voice and acting workshops so as to get, at minimum, a basic understanding of what the actor needs to accomplish in her work. The Alexander coach needs a space for tutorial work that ideally is large enough for an Alexander table[4] and any other standing work the coach may need to do. This normally involves the AT coach working with the actor while the actor is delivering text and helping the actor find her ease. Or the AT coach may just work with the actor in quiet, allowing the actor to make the connections on her own in rehearsal and performance. The good Alexander coach adapts to the actor's individual needs.

Most of the same principles apply to the Alexander coach as the voice/dialect coach: putting notes in a constructive manner; being sensitive to the timing and tone of notes; communicating with the director; maintaining appropriate boundaries with actors

---

[4] Often, Alexander teachers work with an individual while she is lying down, on her back, because this makes it easier for the person to let go of her habits. Usually, the table is a massage table or a table slightly wider and harder than a massage table that is strong enough for someone to lie on. In Alexander world, one calls this *table* or *lying down work*, not to be confused with what we refer to as table work when we sit at a table in rehearsal discussing the details of the text.

and other coaches; and looking for ways to contribute positively to the production.

In some cases, voice coaches are also trained as Alexander coaches, as in my own situation. I have found this provides valuable crossover in terms of how the Alexander principles enhance voice usage. The only time it might prove challenging is if the cast is so large it simply would not be possible for one coach to manage working with everyone, in which case the theater should hire someone whose approach is compatible to work with the assigned voice/dialect/Alexander coach, ideally with the assigned coach's input.

Appreciation

It really helps the coach when the director shows appreciation. Opening night cards help, too!

I coached *The Importance of Being Earnest* at a Shakespeare festival just outside of New York City several years ago. Because of commitments with the Young Company, I was not able to come to rehearsal until a week or so into the rehearsal period. When I came to rehearsal and heard the first run-through, the text was virtually unintelligible. I worked diligently with each actor, gave copious dialect and clarity notes at run-throughs, and, finally, after much hard work, the show became clear. People raved to the director about how funny the show was and how believable the dialect. A British woman in the audience opening night wrote me specifically to say the dialects were so successful that she felt she was back in England. Had the audience members not understood all those jokes, would anyone have been impressed by the production? On opening night, the director, who is also a well-known actor, brought Oscar Wilde t-shirts for the designer, the stage manager, the assistant stage manager, the assistant director, the artistic director, and every actor in the cast. She omitted the vocal/dialect coach. Moral of the story: directors need to remember that the voice/dialect coach's contribution is an integral part of the success of the show. And buy the coach a t-shirt!

In summary, a director can benefit a great deal from working with a voice coach. It behooves the director to collaborate and support the work of the coach as much as she can. In the end, the actors and production will achieve a higher standard and this will reflect well on the director's achievements.

I hope directors will use this book as a guide and that it can be of use to coaches in the rehearsal process. Particular chapters might prove more useful for specific shows and purposes. Certainly, this book should provide a good foundation for students of directing but also for the more experienced director who may have overlooked this important aspect of the theatrical experience.

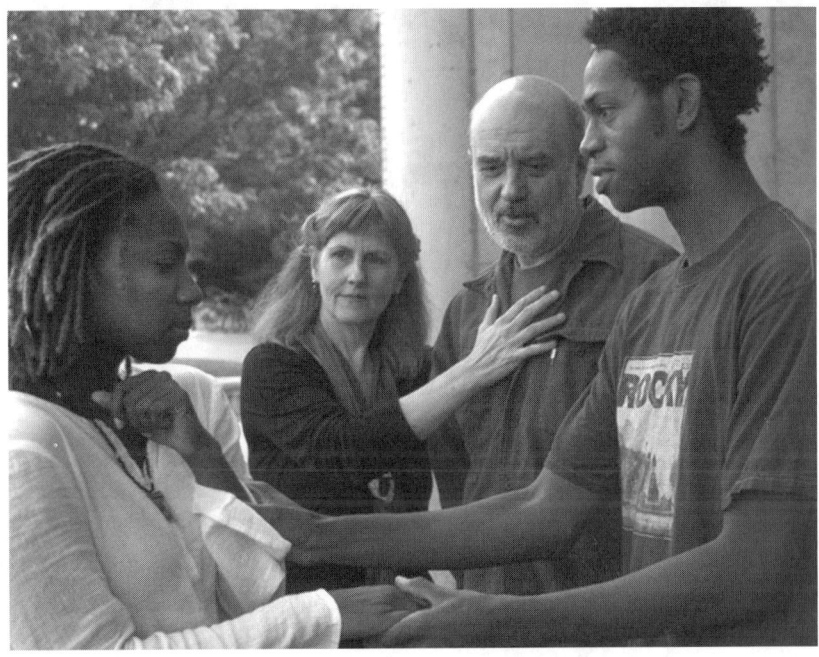

Left to right, Roberta Burke (BFA, Acting, School of Drama, Carnegie Mellon, 2009), Janet Madelle Feindel, (author), Mladen Kiselov (director), and Eric Berryman (BFA, Acting student, School of Drama, Carnegie Mellon). Photo by Karen Waggoner.

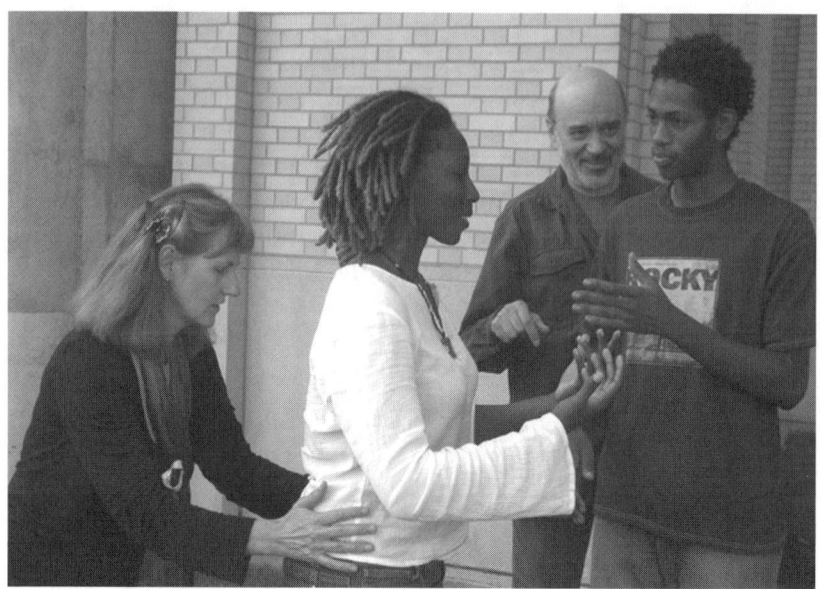

Left to right, Janet Madelle Feindel (author), Roberta Burke (BFA, Acting, School of Drama, Carnegie Mellon, 2009), Mladen Kiselov (director), and Eric Berryman (BFA, Acting student, School of Drama, Carnegie Mellon). Photo by Karen Waggoner.

References

Abraham, F. M. (2005). *A Midsummer Night's Dream: Actors on Shakespeare*. London: Faber & Faber.

Alexander, F. M. (1995). About breathing. In E. Maisel (Ed.), *The Alexander Technique: The essential writings of F. Matthias Alexander* (pp. 41-48). New York: Carol. (Originally published as *The resurrection of the body*.)

Benjamin, B. E., & Sohnen-Moe, C. (2005). *The ethics of touch* (3rd ed.). Tucson, AZ: Sohnen-Moe Associates.

Berry, C. (1973). *Voice and the actor*. Edinburgh, UK: Harrop.

Berry, C. (2000). *The actor and the text*. New York: Applause Books.

Berry, C. (2000). That secret voice. In M. Hampton & B. Acker (Eds.), *The vocal vision: Views on voice by 24 leading teachers, coaches and directors* (pp. 25-35). New York: Applause Books.

Berry, C. (2001). *Text in action*. New York: Virgin Books.

Berry, C. (2008). *From word to play: A textual handbook for actors and directors*. London: Oberon Books.

Bloom, M. (Moderator) (with Diamond, L., Jory, J., Scott, H., & Shapiro, M.). (2002, January). So you want to be a director. *American Theatre Magazine, 1*(19), 26-30, 102-105.

Bruder, M., Cohn, M., Olnek, M., Pollack, N., Previto, R., & Zigler, S. (1986). *A practical handbook for the actor*. Lincolnshire, IL: Vintage.

Carrington, W. (August, 2004). Keynote address presented at the International Congress on the F. M. Alexander Technique. Oxford, England.

Colaianni, L. (1994). *The joy of phonetics and accents*. New York: Drama Publishers.

Colaianni, L., & Anderson, C. (2003). *Bringing speech to life*. New York: Joy Press.

Conable, B. (1995). *How to learn the Alexander Technique: A manual for students*. Portland, OR: Andover Press.

Feindel, J. M. (1986). A particular class of women. In T. Hamill (Ed.), *Singular voices* (pp. 15-155). Toronto, Canada: Canada Playwrights Press.

Gelb, M. (1996). *Body learning: An introduction to the Alexander Technique* (2nd ed.). New York: Holt/Owl Books.

Gilligan, C. (1982). *In a different voice: Psychological theory and women's development.* Cambridge: Harvard University Press.

Goldberg, N. (1986). *Writing down the bones: Freeing the writer within.* Boston: Shambhala.

Goldberg, N. (1990). *Wild mind: Living the writer's life.* New York: Bantam.

Green, R., & Burgess, M. (Writers), & Coulter, A. (Director). (2000). The knight in white satin armor [Television series episode]. In D. Chase (Producer), *The Sopranos.* New York: HBO.

Hampton, M., & Acker, B. (Eds.) (2000). *The vocal vision: Views on voice by 24 leading teachers, coaches and directors.* New York: Applause Books.

Iyengar, B. K. S. (with Evans, J. J., & Abrams, D.). (2005). *Light on life: The yoga journey to wholeness, inner peace, and ultimate freedom.* Emmaus, PA: Rodale.

Knight, D. (2000). Standard speech: The ongoing debate. In M. Hampton & B. Acker (Eds.), *The vocal vision: Views on voice by 24 leading teachers, coaches and directors* (pp. 155-183). New York: Applause Books.

Kohan, J. (Writer), & Seidelman, S. (Director). (1998). The power of female sex [Television series episode]. In D. Star (Producer), *Sex and the City.* New York City: HBO.

Linklater, K. (1976). *Freeing the natural voice.* Hollywood, CA: Drama Publishers.

Linklater, K. (1992). *Freeing Shakespeare's voice.* New York: Theatre Communications Group.

McCallion, M. (1998). *The voice book.* New York: Theatre Arts Books/ Routledge.

McEvenue, K. (2002). *The actor and the Alexander Technique.* Basingstoke, UK: Palgrave Macmillan.

McLean, M. P. (1968). *Good American speech.* New York: Dutton.

Shurtleff, M. (2003). *Audition: Everything an actor needs to know to get the part.* New York: Walker & Company.

Skinner, E. W. (1990). *Speak with distinction.* (Rev. ed.). New York: Applause Books.

Truth, S. (1851). Ain't I a woman?

Williams, T. (1947). *A streetcar named desire.* New York: New Directions Books.

Williamson, M. (1992). *Return to love.* New York: Harper Collins.

Winter, T. (Writer), & Van Patten, T. (Director). (2002). House arrest [Television series episode]. In D. Chase (Producer), *The Sopranos.* New York: HBO.

Zito, R. (June, 1999). Workshop presented at Care of the Professional Voice Symposium, Acting Voice. Philadelphia, PA.

Zito, R. (June, 2000). Workshop presented at Care of the Professional Voice Symposium, Acting Voice. Philadelphia, PA.

Resources

INDEX TO RESOURCES

Accents and Dialects	193
Alexander Technique	195
Anatomy	198
Education, Creativity, and Psychology	199
Speech	200
Tongue Twisters	201
Vocal Health	201
Voice	205
Other Organizations Related to Voice, Acting, and Directing	208

ACCENTS AND DIALECTS

Blumenfeld, R. (1998). *Accents: A manual for actors.* New York: Limelight Editions.

A thorough manual covering a wide variety of dialects. The accompanying CD is useful although he speaks extremely quickly without time to repeat words and phrases. Reader is advised to also use examples of native speakers.

Blunt, J. (1984). *Stage dialects.* Woodstock, IL: Dramatic Publishing.

Particularly useful for dialects of the British Isles, Blunt's book includes useful drills and accompanying tapes on which Blunt reads the drills and provides samples of native speakers.

Ferry, D., & Smukler, D., & Canajun, E. (2000). *Canadian dialects for actors*. Independently produced by David Ferry.

An excellent CD covering accents in Canada from coast to coast, presented as a series of monologues. Soon they will be publishing an accompanying book.

Gimson, A. C. (1964). *An introduction to the pronunciation of English*. London: Edward Arnold.

Herman, L. (1997). *Foreign dialects: A manual for actors, directors and writers*. New York: Routledge.

Hughes, A., & Trudgill, P. (1983). *English accents and dialects* (3rd ed.). London: Edward Arnold.

International Dialects of English Archive (IDEA) Web site

An excellent Web site with various examples and guidelines for many dialects and accents.

http://web.ku.edu/idea/
Professor Paul Meier, Founder and Director (pmeier@ku.edu)
Shawn M. Muller, Webmaster and Technical Director (shawnmuller@earthlink.net)
Address:
IDEA
Professor Paul Meier, Director
Theatre and Film Department
University of Kansas
Lawrence, KS, 66045 USA
Phone: (785) 864-2692
Fax: (785) 864-5251

Paul Meier also offers a well-organized and thorough book and accompanying CD, with a solid approach to accent and dialect for the actor, Accents and Dialects for Stage and Screen *(Paul Meier Dialect Services, 4316 Wimbledon Drive, Lawrence, Kansas, 66047, USA*; http://www.paulmeier.com).

Kopf, G. (2005). *The dialect handbook*. Orlando, FL: Voiceprint Publishing.

Kur, B. (2000). *Stage dialect studies*. Available through the author: 609 West Fairmount Avenue, State College, PA 16801.

Lane-Plescia, G. Dialects and accents for actors. A variety of CDs available from http://www.dialectresource.com/index.html

These CDs offer a great range of dialects and accents with practical suggestions in terms of sound changes and rhythm changes, with examples of native speakers. The examples of native speakers are not recorded in a studio setting, so the reader is advised to supplement with other sources.

Machlin, E. (2006). *Dialects for the stage.* New York: Theatre Arts Books.

Molin, D. H. (1991). *Actor's encyclopedia of dialects* (2nd ed.). New York: Sterling Publishers.

Stern, D. A. *Acting with an accent.* Lyndonville, VT: Dialect Accents Specialists. A series of accent CDs available from Dialect Accents Specialists, Inc., 51 Depot St. Lyndonville, VT 05851-0044, http://www.dialectaccentspecialists.com/store/

Stern's approach includes useful tips about the "point of focus" and resonance of different accents and dialects. In general, his work is most useful for American dialects. His work should be supplemented with examples of native speakers and other approaches, particularly for the European accents and dialects.

Wells, J. C. (1985). *Accents of English.* London: Cambridge University Press.

ALEXANDER TECHNIQUE

Texts

Barker, S. (1978). *The Alexander Technique: The revolutionary way to use your body for total energy.* New York: Bantam Books.

A clear and basic introduction to the Alexander Technique. Barker is also a teacher of movement for the theater and has taught at various professional training programs, including Shakespeare & Company.

Barlow, W. (2001). *The Alexander principle: How to use your body without stress*. London: Orion Books.

Wilfred Barlow, who trained with F. M. Alexander, was also a qualified medical doctor. He approaches the technique from a scientific and medical viewpoint, considering many aspects of the application of the technique in the areas of physical and mental health.

Carrington, W. (2004). *Thinking aloud: Talks on teaching the Alexander Technique*. Berkeley, CA: Mornum Time Press.

Carrington writes short chapters, each dealing with specific issues around application of the Alexander Technique. Carrington was one of the Alexander teachers trained by F. M. Alexander himself. He wrote this originally for teachers although interested laypersons have found the book useful as well.

Gelb, M. (1996). *Body learning: An introduction to the Alexander Technique*. New York: Holt/Owl Books.

This is an excellent introduction to the basics of the Alexander Technique for the beginning student.

Heirich, J. (2005). *Voice and the Alexander Technique*. San Francisco: Mornum Time Press.

This book deals primarily with the Alexander Technique as it relates to the singing voice, drawing on the author's many years of teaching experience.

Jones, F. P. (1997). *Freedom to change: The development and science of the Alexander Technique*. London: Mouritz.

Jones draws on his years researching the Alexander Technique and offers scientific support for the principles of the technique. He discusses in depth his long association with F. M. Alexander, with interesting biographical material.

Langford, E. (1999). *Mind and muscle, an owner's manual*. Leuven, Belgium: Garant Publishing.

A clear explanation of the Alexander Technique. Langford trained with Walter Carrington and is a musician. (Langford also wrote Only connect: Reflections on teaching the Alexander Technique *(2004), which is also an excellent book on how one communicates about the technique, geared toward teachers of the Alexander Technique.)*

McDonald, G. (1998). *Alexander Technique: A practical program for health, poise and fitness.* Alexandria, Va.: Time-Life Books.

Maisel, E. (Ed.) (2000). *The Alexander Technique: The essential writings of F. M. Alexander.* New York: Citadel.
This is an excellent foundation book for the Alexander Technique. It includes Alexander's most comprehensible writing on various applications of the technique.

McEvenue, K. (2002). *The actor and the Alexander Technique.* Basingstoke, UK: Palgave Macmillan.
This book deals with how to apply the technique in practical ways in rehearsal and performance situations. McEvenue draws on her extensive experience working with professional actors and directors, primarily at the Stratford Shakespeare Festival, Canada.

Oppenheimer, A. (Ed.). (2005). *The congress papers, exploring the principles.* London: Society of Teachers of the Alexander Technique Books.
These papers are based on lectures and workshops of the International Congress on the F. M. Alexander Technique held in Oxford, UK, with articles by some of the world's top Alexander teachers, including Walter Carrington. Also included is an article on voice for Alexander teachers by the author, Janet Madelle Feindel, MFA. Another collection of the Congress Papers from the congress, held in 2008 in Lugano, Switzerland, due in 2009, edited by Jean Fischer, also includes an article by the author.

Alexander Technique Organizations

The Alexander Alliance
The Alexander Alliance, founded by Bruce Fertman and Martha Hansen-Fertman, offers teacher training programs around the world.
http://www.alexanderalliance.com/

Alexander Technique International (ATI)

ATI functions as an information source about Alexander teachers, provides workshops and training programs worldwide, and produces a journal several times a year. The Web site also provides information about publications and issues related to the Alexander Technique. ATI also acts as a certifying body for Alexander teachers.

United States (Main Office):
Linda Hein, Administrative Assistant
E-mail: ati-usa@ati-net.com
1692 Massachusetts Ave., 3rd floor
Cambridge, MA 02138, USA
Telephone: 888-668-8996 (toll-free from Canada and USA)
617-497-5151
Fax: 617-497-2615

Other offices worldwide available on the Web site
http://www.ati-net.com/

American Society for the Alexander Technique (AmSAT)
http://www.alexandertech.org/

Society of Teachers of the Alexander Technique (STAT)

The mother organization of CanSTAT, AmSTAT, and other national certifying bodies for Alexander teachers. Their Web site includes information about the technique, workshops, training programs, and publications. STAT also publishes the papers of the International Congress, which occurs every 4 years.

http://www.stat.org.uk/

ANATOMY

Hale, R. B., & Coyle, T. (1988). *Albinus on anatomy*. New York: Dover Publications.

Basic anatomy useful for movement studies.

Miller, J. (1983). *The human body*. Northampton, UK: Viking Press.

This pop-up anatomy book is excellent for understanding vocal mechanisms and anatomy.

Netter, F. (2006). *Atlas of the human body* (4th ed.). Amsterdam, Netherlands: Saunders, Elsevier.

Contains wonderfully detailed color pictures of the diaphragm from a variety of angles, intercostal muscles both internal and external, and the muscles of the neck and back, useful for understanding the Alexander technique.

Takahashi, T. (1989). *Atlas of the human body*. Tokyo: Kodansha.

Contains particularly good color pictures of the respiratory system and especially the diaphragm for its full width.

Vannini, V. (1981). *The color atlas of human anatomy*. New York: Harmony Books.

Contains excellent pictures of diaphragm and breath apparatus, as well as the larynx and pharynx (throat).

EDUCATION, CREATIVITY, AND PSYCHOLOGY

Benjamin, B. E., & Sohnen-Moe, C. (2005). *The ethics of touch* (3rd ed.). Tucson, AZ: Sohnen-Moe Associates.

An excellent source book designed primarily for massage therapists but also a useful source for voice and Alexander teachers.

Cameron, J. (1992). *The artist's way*. New York: G. P. Putnam's Sons.

Spiritual and psychological connection to art; explorations to aid in self-discovery; numerous quotes about art and spirituality.

McIntosh, N. (2005). *The educated heart: Professional boundaries for massage therapists, bodyworkers, and movement teachers.* Philadelphia: Lippincott Williams & Wilkins.

This book is particularly useful for voice and Alexander coaches to help clarify roles and boundaries in the often-challenging situations that coaches find themselves in working in the theater, training programs, and media.

Palmer, P. (1998). *The courage to teach: Exploring the landscape of a teacher's life.* Hoboken, NJ: Jossey-Bass Publishers.

Although this book is not related to theater directly in any way, it is included because it identifies so exquisitely the spiritual goals in teaching and is completely applicable to coaching, acting, and directing.

Rosen, D. C, & Sataloff, R. T. (1997). *Psychology of voice disorders.* San Diego, CA: Singular Press.

Deals with various therapeutic issues for the professional voice user.

SPEECH

Colaianni, L. (1994). *The joy of phonetics and accents.* New York: Drama Publishers.

A descriptive and kinesthetic approach to speech that explores the International Phonetic Alphabet and includes exercises using phonetic pillows to teach speech, dialects, and accents.

Colaianni, L., & Anderson, C. (2003). *Bringing speech to life.* New York: Joy Press.

A workbook to accompany The Joy of Phonetics *and useful for training of actors and directors.*

Skinner, E., Monich, T., & Mansell, L. (1991). *Speak with distinction.* New York: Applause Books.

An introduction to Standard American Speech and Skinner's Phonetic Alphabet, complete with drills and text selections.

The Voice and Speech Trainers Association (VASTA) & Dal Vera, R. (2001). *The voice in violence.* New York: Applause Books.

Deals with techniques to enable performers to perform violence without vocal damage.

The Voice and Speech Trainers Association (VASTA), Dal Vera, R., & Colaianni, L. (2001). *Standard speech: Essays on voice and speech.* New York: Applause Books.

Explores controversy around issues in speech pedagogy.

TONGUE TWISTERS

Karshner, R. (1993). *You said a mouthful.* Rancho Mirage, CA: DramaLine Books.

Good tongue twisters organized alphabetically.

Parkin, K. (1969). *Tongue twisters.* New York: Samuel French.

Good, old-fashioned tongue twisters organized according to sound requirements, but check them first as some are definitely not politically correct.

VOCAL HEALTH

Benninger, M., & Murry, T. (2006). *The performer's voice.* San Diego, CA: Plural Publishing.

Discusses treatment for dealing with voice care, primarily medical, with chapters by Jean Abitbol, MD, a chapter from the singer's perspective by Jeannette Lovetri, and an acting voice perspective by J. M. Feindel, MFA.

Sataloff, R. T. (1991). *Professional voice: The science and art of clinical care.* San Diego, CA: Singular Publishing.

A basic medical overview with an explanation of voice disorders and color illustrations.

Sataloff, R. T. (2006). *Vocal health and pedagogy: Advanced assessment and treatment* (2nd ed.). San Diego, CA: Plural Publishing.

An excellent overview of interdisciplinary voice care from both medical and artistic perspectives.

(*NOTE:* **Plural Publishing offers many books, CDs, and tapes on voice production, vocal anatomy, and voice health.**)

Singing Journal

Published by the National Association of Singing Teachers, this is a regular publication on singing, singing pedagogy, and voice care.

Voice and Speech Trainers Association Newsletter and Journals

Contain articles on voice care and listings of events, conferences, and training workshops.

Voice Journal

Published by the Voice Foundation, this is a regular publication on voice medicine and research.

Voice

Texts

Barton, R. (with Dal Vera, R.). (1995). *Voice: Onstage and off.* Lewisville, TX: Harcourt Brace.

A useful voice book dealing with challenges for the actor in a number of performance situations.

Berry, C. (1973). *Voice and the actor.* Edinburgh, UK: Harrop.

Deals with foundation in voice production with many text examples, and is the basis for most voice training in drama schools in the United Kingdom as well as internationally.

Berry, C. (2000). *The actor and the text.* New York: Applause Books.

This book is a classic for directors, voice coaches, and actors, and includes in-depth work and practical exercises for examining the connection of voice and text as well as approaching text analysis.

Berry, C. (2001). *Text in action.* New York: Virgin Books.

This book is based on Berry's work with directors and the director's workshops she led through Theatre for a New Audience in New York City. Essential for directors and directing students.

Berry, C. (2008). *From word to play: A textual handbook for actors and directors.* London: Oberon Books.

This book delves more deeply into the process of bringing the text alive in a rehearsal process, based on Berry's far-ranging work at the Royal Shakespeare Company and Theatre for a New Audience, among others.

Cook, J. (1980). *Women in Shakespeare.* Edinburgh, UK: Harrop.

A study of actresses who performed Shakespeare from the 1960s to 1980 in England.

Hampton, M., & Acker, B. (Eds.). (2000). *The vocal vision: Views on voice by 24 leading teachers, coaches and directors.* New York: Applause Books.

A collection of essays including Catherine Fitzmaurice's article "Breathing is meaning" and other articles related to voice pedagogy, controversial issues in teaching, and various techniques.

Houfek, N. (Edited by Watson, L., & de Vries, L.) (2001). *How to use a vocal coach: A practical guide for directors.* Retrieved February 25, 2009, from http://www.vasta.org.

Also includes a list of other pertinent articles written by VASTA members Bonnie Raphael, Ralph Zito, and others.

Lecky, W. S. (2007). *Vox method: Training the voice.* Montreal: Centre Collégial de Développement de Matériel Didactique.

Extremely thorough training method with DVD for college-level acting students. Lecky chairs the theater program at Dawson College in Montreal, Canada.

Lessac, A. (1997). *The use and training of the human voice.* New York: McGraw-Hill.

This book clearly outlines the Lessac approach to voice training, comparing the human sounds of the voice to various aspects of an orchestra. The classic ybuzz call *and other aspects of his approach are clearly detailed.*

Linklater, K. (1976). *Freeing the natural voice.* New York: Drama Publishers.

Basic introduction to the Linklater approach to voice work—the original edition of Kristin Linklater's book.

Linklater, K. (1992). *Freeing Shakespeare's voice: The actor's guide to talking the text.* New York: Theatre Communications Group.

Explorations of voice/text and psychophysical work using the Linklater approach to the work as the foundation for the explorations.

Linklater, K. (2006). *Freeing the natural voice: Imagery and art in the practice of voice and language.* New York: Drama Publishers.

This revised edition of Linklater's method, used in drama schools throughout the United States and internationally for the last 30 years, provides a clear overview of her method, with added emphasis on the use of imagery and imagination in developing the voice. A valuable supplement to the first edition.

Martin, J. (1991). *The voice in modern theatre.* New York: Routledge.

The history of new approaches to voice in the 20th century; concentrates more on British than American trainers; good overview.

McCallion, M. (1998). *The voice book.* New York: Theatre Arts Books/Routledge.

Explores many aspects of voice/speech/text with practical tips for adapting voice use for specific situations in theater, film voice-over, etc. The late McCallion has incorporated the principles of the Alexander Technique with the voice overview in a particularly effective manner.

Melton, J. (with Tom, K.) (2000). *One voice: Integrating singing technique and theatre voice training.* Portsmouth, NH: Heinemann Drama.

Melton is a master Fitzmaurice voice teacher, New York City voice coach, and a singing specialist, who has taught internationally. This is a terrific book for directors of musical theater who need to understand the organic connection of the speaking and singing voice.

Rodenburg, P. (1993). *The right to speak: Working with the voice.* New York: Theatre Arts Books.

Basic vocal approach; deals with the voice as it relates to the "right to express" and self-image in our society and particularly useful as a training tool for actors.

Rodenburg, P. (1994). *The need for words.* New York: Theatre Arts Book.

More voice/text explorations and extremely useful for directors as well as actors.

Rodenburg, P. (2000). *The actor speaks: Voice and the performer.* New York: St. Martin's Press.

Deals with voice curriculum and vocal demands in various performance situations.

Shakespeare, W., & Freeman, N. (Ed.) *Applause First Folio Editions.* New York, London: Applause Books.

Numerous books on working with Shakespeare's first folio. Freeman worked with Shakespeare & Company and the Voice Intensive at Simon Fraser. Also see http://www.neilfreeman.com.

Withers-Wilson, N. (1993). *Vocal direction for the theater.* New York: Drama Books.

An overview of a voice coach's responsibilities; some history of voice training in America; voice and the rehearsal process.

VOICE

Additional Voice Resources

The British Voice Association

The association's mission is to encourage healthy voices, vocal skills, and communication in performing arts, business, and industry, with a focus on medicine and education dealing with voice difficulties ranging from severe pathology and cancer to more nuanced challenges in artistic performance.

The Canadian Voice Care Foundation
Chairwoman: Katherine Ardo

Promotes interdisciplinary exchange of information and sponsors symposia. The Canadian Voice Care Symposium leans more toward pedagogical aspects of voice, along with clinical aspects of voice care; generally includes several master classes both in speaking voice and singing voice.

2828 Toronto Crescent NW
Calgary, Alberta, Canada
T2N 3W2
Telephone: 403-284-9590

Jo Estill Web Site

This Web site provides an overview of training concepts, history, listing of teachers, and available courses.

http://www.trainmyvoice.com/

Fitzmaurice Voice Teachers Web site

Overview of Fitzmaurice work, updates on international workshops, information about training programs and how to find a Fitzmaurice teacher in one's area.

http://www.fitzmauricevoice.com/about.htm

Roy Hart Center, France

Provides workshops, information about Roy Hart teachers, and training for certification in the Roy Hart voice work.

http://www.roy-hart.com

Arthur Lessac Training and Research Institute

The institute offers training and teacher training programs. The Web site provides an overview of the approach, listing of teachers, courses, etc.

http://www.lessacinstitute.com/bio.html

Linklater Voice Teachers Web site

Kristin Linklater's Web site with information on her books, many articles, international listing of teachers, and information about training programs and how to locate designated Linklater teachers.

http://www.kristinlinklater.com/

Pacific Voice Care Foundation
Chairman: Dr. K. Izdebski

An annual voice symposium held on the West Coast with international faculty of interdisciplinary voice specialists.

350 Parnassus #501
San Francisco, CA 94117

Voice and Speech Trainers Association (VASTA)

An organization for voice and speech trainers, providing information on members, workshops, newsletter, and publishing The Voice and Speech Review. *On their Web site one can find listings of voice teachers in specific areas of North America and their training.*

http://www.vasta.org

Voice Clinic through the University of Pittsburgh, with Dr. Clark Rosen, Dr. Stephen Buckmire (both laryngologists), Dr. Katherine Verdolini (speech pathologist), but as yet no voice/speech trainer
University of Pittsburgh Voice Center
Department of Otolaryngology
200 Lothrop Street
Pittsburgh, PA 15215
Telephone: 412-647-2112

The Voice Foundation, USA
Chairman: Dr. Robert Sataloff

An organization encouraging interdisciplinary work among voice and speech trainers, speech pathologists, singing teachers, laryngologists, acoustic specialists, and ear, nose, and throat specialists along with other related fields such as teachers of the Alexander and Feldenkrais methods. Sponsors the annual Care of the

Professional Voice Symposium, an interdisciplinary conference leaning heavily on the scientific research aspects of voice care but also including some practical workshops and master classes in singing voice.

Interdisciplinary voice clinic in Philadelphia:
1721 Pine Street
Philadelphia, PA 19103
Telephone: 215-735-7999
http://voicefoundation.org

OTHER ORGANIZATIONS RELATED TO VOICE, ACTING, AND DIRECTING

Actors Equity
http://www.actorsequity.org

American Speech-Language-Hearing Association (ASHA)
http://www.asha.org

Association of Teachers of Singing (AOTOS)
http://www.aotos.co.uk

British Actors Equity
http://www.equity.org.uk/

British Association for Performing Arts Medicine (BAPAM)
http://www.bapam.org.uk

British Association of Otolaryngology (BAOL)
http://www.entuk.org

Canadian Actors Equity (also deals with contracts for stage directors)
http://www.caea.com

Directors Guild of America
http://www.dga.org

Directors Guild of Great Britain
4 Windmill Street
London, UK
WIT 2 HZ
http://www.dggb.co.uk/

Incorporated Society of Musicians (ISM)
http://www.ism.org

International Association of Logopedics and Phoniatrics (IALP)
http://www.ialp.info

International Federation of Oto-Rhino-Laryngological Societies (IFOS)
http://www.ifosworld.org

Musicians Union
http://www.musiciansunion.org.uk

National Association of Teachers of Singing (NATS)
http://www.nats.org

National Center for Voice and Speech—A Division of The Denver Center for the Performing Arts, Denver, Colorado, USA
http://www.ncvs.org

Royal College of Speech and Language Therapists (RCSLT)
http://www.rcslt.org

Voice Care Network
http://www.voicecare.org.uk

Voluntary Arts Network
http://www.voluntaryarts.org

World Voice Day (American Academy of Otolaryngology—Head and Neck Surgery)
www.entnet.org

APPENDIX

Anatomy and Physiology of the Voice

The voice is similar to any other musical instrument that one might play. As a musician sits down to play an instrument, the quality of the performance is impacted both by how the instrument is maintained and how it is used. The situation is similar for the human voice. There are numerous ways in which we can safeguard the vocal mechanism's structures and function, even independent of how we use the voice. There are also issues of skill that influence voice output. Just a subtle change in the actor's voice can present a challenge for the actor relying on a high level of performance from his instrument. An actor's failure to execute certain vocal gestures can detract from a director's vision for a piece of theater. Accordingly, to elicit optimal results from actors, directors may benefit from an understanding of the vocal mechanism. This Appendix provides the director with an overview of the anatomy and physiology of the vocal mechanism as well as suggestions for achieving healthy and effective vocal expression in the short and long term. A reference list indicating sources for the information in the Appendix as well as further reading is included at the end of the Appendix.

Anatomy of the Larynx

Hard Structures of the Larynx

The human voice is the result of the interaction among many anatomical production units. The larynx, colloquially known as the "voice box," is located within the neck (Figure A-1) and consists of several cartilaginous structures and a single bone (Figure A-2).

One structure that serves to protect the vocal folds—the paired tissues that vibrate to produce sound—is the thyroid cartilage (cartilage is a tough, elastic tissue found in the nose, throat, ear, and other parts of the body). The thyroid cartilage consists of two laminae (or "plates") that join at an angle in the front of the neck but remain open posteriorly (situated near or toward the back

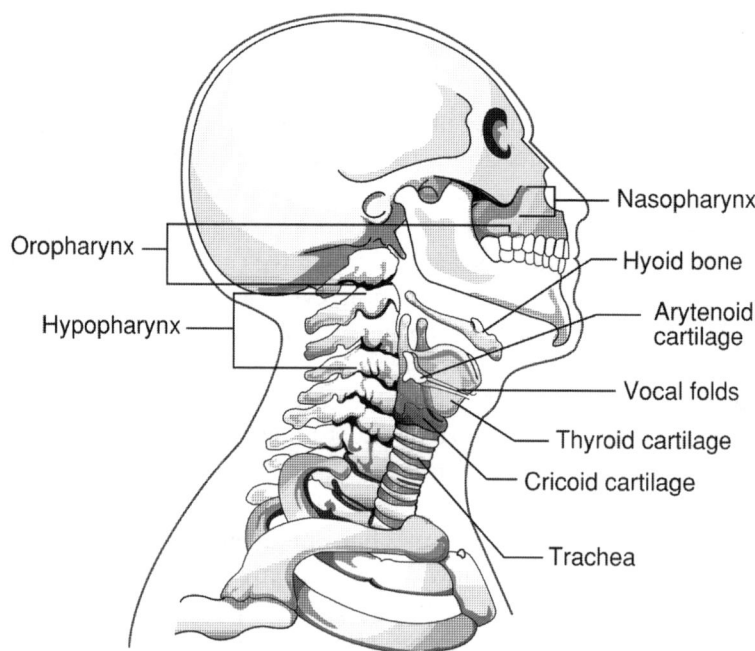

Figure A-1. Larynx in relation to head and neck. Adapted from *The Larynx: A Multidisciplinary Approach* (2nd ed., p. 34), by M. P. Fried, 1996, Philadelphia: Mosby. Adapted with permission.

ANATOMY AND PHYSIOLOGY OF THE VOICE 213

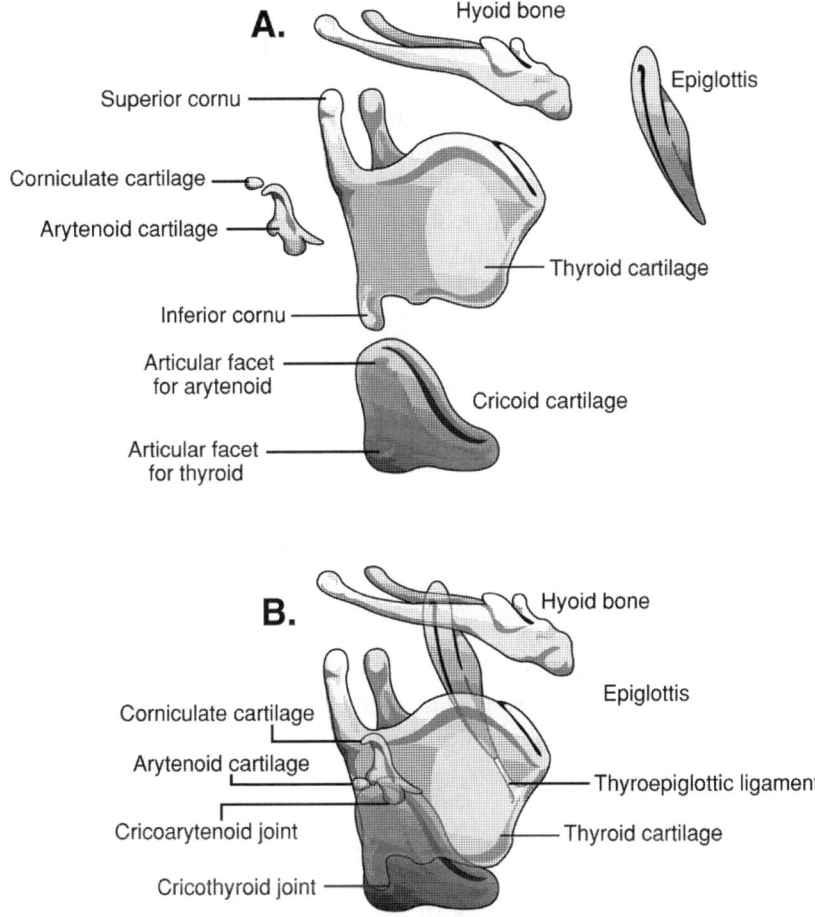

Figure A-2. Hard tissue of the larynx. Adapted from *The Larynx: A Multidisciplinary Approach* (2nd ed., p. 35), by M. P. Fried, 1996, Philadelphia: Mosby. Adapted with permission.

of the body). The point at which the two laminae join is known as the laryngeal prominence. The prominence, popularly known as the "Adam's apple," can be easily seen on a man, but can also be identified on a woman. The thyroid cartilage also serves as a point of attachment for the anterior (situated at or near the front of the body) portion of the vocal folds. This attachment is called the anterior commissure.

The thyroid cartilage sits atop the cricoid cartilage. The cricoid cartilage is a completely circular piece of cartilage that is positioned at the top of the trachea, and is indeed the first ring of the trachea. Resting on the posterior part of the cricoid cartilage are two arytenoid cartilages. Each arytenoid is a pyramidal piece of cartilage that swivels and rocks to adduct (move the vocal folds from an open position to a closed position) the vocal folds during voice production or swallowing and abduct (moving the vocal folds from a closed to an open position) the vocal folds during breathing. Another cartilaginous structure of the larynx is the epiglottis. It is a leaflike structure that attaches to the inside surface of the thyroid cartilage just above the anterior commissure. The epiglottis certainly plays a role in swallowing by covering the airway during swallowing (Ardran & Kemp, 1956). There is evidence that the epiglottis can also affect voice production. Specifically, when the epiglottis is positioned toward the posterior pharyngeal wall, it creates a narrow cavity that can resonate (amplify) high-frequency acoustic energy produced by the vocal folds during voicing, and thus is one source of the brilliant "ring" in a speaker's or singer's voice (Sundberg, 1977). The last major hard structure in the larynx is the hyoid bone, resting slightly above the thyroid cartilage, and serving as a point of attachment for muscles and membranes above and below it.

Laryngeal Musculature

The larynx contains two sets of muscles called the intrinsic and extrinsic muscles. The intrinsic muscles of the larynx are muscles that connect the individual laryngeal structures to one another. Therefore, these muscles are contained within the larynx. The extrinsic muscles of the larynx are muscles that connect the laryngeal structures with structures that are outside of the larynx. These muscles have points of attachment within the larynx as well as to the surrounding structures.

Extrinsic Muscles of the Larynx

The larynx is suspended in a complex of muscles called the extrinsic laryngeal muscles that maintain the larynx's position in the neck at rest and also aid in raising and lowering it during specific functions. The extrinsic musculature can be divided into suprahyoid and infrahyoid muscles. Suprahyoid muscles originate at the larynx either through an attachment to the hyoid bone or the thyroid cartilage, and insert at a point above the larynx. These muscles play a role in elevating the larynx. For instance, as one produces a higher pitch, the larynx generally rises. Similarly, the larynx rises during the first part of a swallow (Ardran & Kemp, 1956). The rise can be visualized by an upward movement of the laryngeal prominence. Infrahyoid muscles originate at the larynx and insert below it. Yawning is a behavior during which the infrahyoid muscles contract. The larynx lowers during this action. In general, the larynx should be allowed to move freely during voice production. If an actor demonstrates excess tension in the extrinsic laryngeal muscles the larynx may be "stuck" in the neck. Activation of the suprahyoid muscles, for instance, will tend to pull the larynx up so that it is positioned high in the neck. This positioning will impact the quality of the voice.

Intrinsic Muscles of the Larynx

A set of muscles called the intrinsic musculature is directly responsible for the production of voice, or *phonation* (Figure A-3).

The main muscle underlying the vibratory tissues of the vocal folds is called the thyroarytenoid muscle (TA). This paired muscle spans from the vocal process of the arytenoid cartilage to the anterior commissure. Two other paired intrinsic muscles, the lateral cricoarytenoid (LCA) and interarytenoid (IA) muscles, are responsible for adducting the vocal folds. When these muscles contract, they draw the arytenoids together and, as a result, bring the TA toward midline. Additionally, the LCA maintains medial compression whereas the IA brings the posterior portion of the TA together. The posterior cricoarytenoid muscle (PCA) abducts the vocal folds during ventilation.

Finally, the cricothyroid muscle (CT) rocks the thyroid cartilage forward—or rocks the cricoid cartilage up and backwards—so that the vocal folds elongate. When the vocal folds are elongated, the *mucosa* overlying the folds (discussed below) is stretched, and its intrinsic stiffness is increased. The result is an increase in the frequency of mucosal vibration during phonation, and thus an increase in what we perceive as pitch. As such, the CT is the main muscle

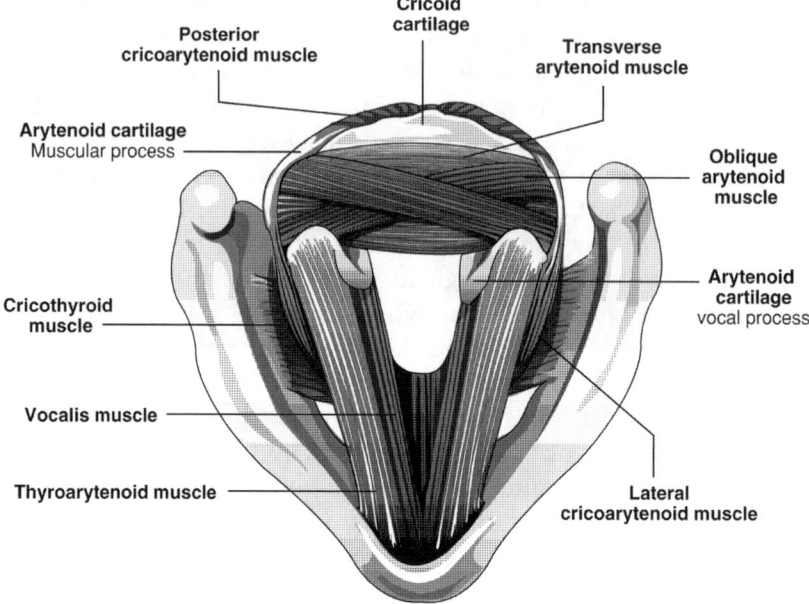

Figure A-3. Intrinsic muscles of the larynx. Adapted from *Atlas of Human Anatomy* (p. 79), 2001, Springhouse, PA: Springhouse Corporation. Adapted with permission.

responsible for increasing pitch. However, it is thought that a section of the PCA, the lateral (vertical) belly, is also important for pitch because it helps to stabilize the arytenoid cartilages when the CT pulls the vocal folds forward (Bryant et al., 1996). Without such stabilization, the CT's ability to stretch the vocal folds would be limited.

Layers of the Vocal Fold

The vocal fold consists of several layers of tissue (Figure A-4). The outermost or superficial layer is called the epithelium. Not only in the vocal folds but also in other tissues, the epithelium, which is formed by epithelial cells, is thin and separates the body from the external environment. This barrier is thus the body's first line of defense in protecting tissue from foreign substances. As a result, the epithelium is quite susceptible to damage. In the vocal folds, the epithelium comprises several layers of *squamous* cells, which

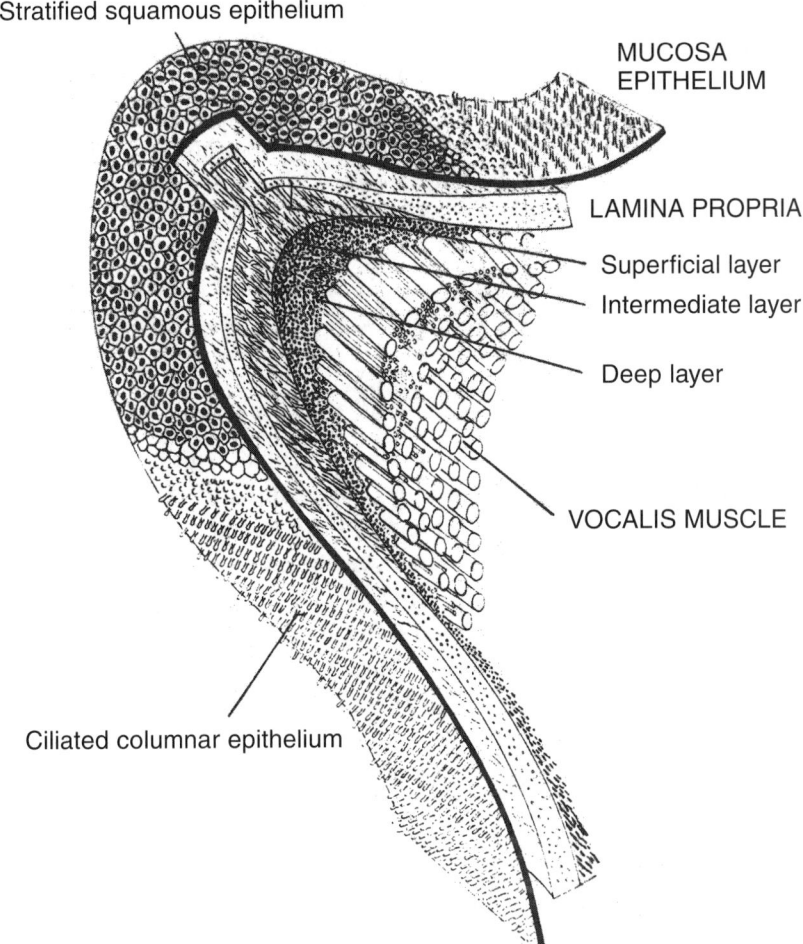

Figure A-4. Layers of the vocal fold. From "Phonosurgery—Basic and Clinical Investigations," by M. Hirano, 1975, *Otologia (Fukuoka)*, *21*, p. 241. Reprinted with permission.

are cubic in shape. The base of the epithelium is formed by what is called the basement membrane zone (Gray, Pignatari, & Harding, 1994). Tiny anchoring fibers extend from this region into the next layer of tissue—the superficial lamina propria—securing the adherence of the layers. Functionally, the epithelium and superficial lamina propria are coupled and together are called the mucosa. The next two layers of the vocal fold are the intermediate and deep layers of the lamina propria. These two layers consist of varying amounts of collagen and elastin fibers (Hammond, Gray, & Butler, 2000; Hammond, Gray, Butler, Zhou, & Hammond, 1998; Tateya, Tateya, & Bless, 2006). The vocal ligament is a term that refers to these two layers as a unit. The TA muscle is the innermost layer of the vocal fold and is composed of contractile muscle fibers.

Breathing Physiology

Inhalation

Inhalation and exhalation are obviously crucial aspects of phonation. Inhalation refers to the process of moving air from outside the body into the lungs. This happens with the coordination of several muscular actions. First, the diaphragm, a skeletal muscle that attaches to the base of the lungs and extends across the body front to back, contracts, and, in doing so, lowers. Because of its location, we cannot see the contraction of the diaphragm directly (Figure A-5).

However, we can infer that the diaphragm has contracted and descended because it pushes against the contents of the abdomen,

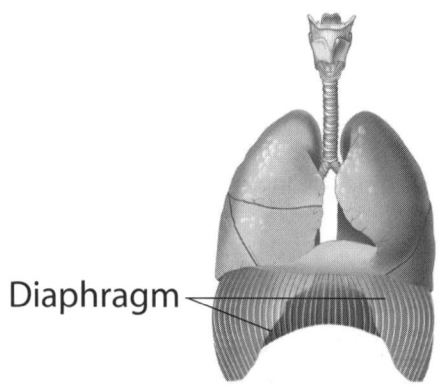

Figure A-5. Diaphragm. Adapted from *The Vocal Instrument* (p. 11), by S. Radionoff, 2008, San Diego, CA: Plural Publishing. Copyright 2008. Adapted with permission.

which are waterlike and cannot be compressed. Therefore, when the diaphragm lowers, the abdomen distends outward. Because of the attachment between the diaphragm and the lungs, when the diaphragm lowers, the lungs are pulled down and their volume is increased in the vertical dimension. Other muscles also contract during inhalation. Muscles between the ribs, known as the external intercostals, contract and pull the ribs up and out. Because the ribs are attached to the lungs, expansion of the ribcage causes the lungs to expand equivalently. When lung volume increases in any dimension—due to diaphragmatic or rib muscle contractions—the pressure inside them is decreased. As a result, the air pressure within the lungs becomes less than the air pressure of the environment. Air, as water, tends to flow from regions of higher pressure to regions of lower pressure, and, as a result, air rushes into the lungs. Air enters through the nose or mouth, and then passes into the pharynx, through the larynx, down the trachea, and finally fills the lungs.

Exhalation

Exhalation is the process of air moving from within the lungs to outside the body. This process occurs because the lungs compress, increasing the air pressure inside them, which now becomes greater than the air pressure in the environment. Lung compression can occur by way of several different mechanisms. First, once the lungs have been expanded during prior inhalation, the stretched lungs-ribcage unit demonstrates a recoil force to return to its original resting position. This tendency is due to the elasticity of the tissue. Just as a rubber band generates a force in the direction of its original resting state after being stretched, similarly the coupled lungs-ribcage unit generates a force in the direction of their resting state when they are distorted away from it. Thus, at the same time as muscular inspiratory forces are reduced at the end of inhalation, the lungs-ribcage unit will tend to collapse to its resting position, thus reducing the lungs' dimensions. Second, muscular forces during expiration often further add to lung compression. Typically, the diaphragm slowly relaxes. The resulting upward movement of the diaphragm helps to return the lungs to their preexpansion state. Similarly, rib muscles called the internal intercostals contract and reduce ribcage dimensions, and with it the dimensions of the lungs.

Finally, abdominal and back muscles contract. As noted, the contents of the abdomen are waterlike, and as such are not compressible. When the abdominal and back muscles contract—especially the deep transverse muscle, which is similar to a girdle around the lower part of the torso—the abdominal contents are displaced. The only direction for them to displace is upwards, pushing the diaphragm up and with it decreasing the vertical dimension of the lungs. As a result of these forces, pressure inside the lungs is increased relative to atmospheric pressure and air tends to flow from this high-pressure region to the lower pressure region outside the body.

PHONATORY PHYSIOLOGY

The vocal folds vibrate when air flows through the glottis, the space between the vocal folds. This process is known as phonation. For speech, phonation typically occurs during the exhalatory phase of ventilation. For phonation to occur, first, the PCA muscles contract and abduct the vocal folds in order for air to be inhaled. Once air has entered the lungs, the IA, LCA, and TA muscles contract and adduct the vocal folds.

The exhalation process begins at about the same time, as described previously. Air molecules build up under the closed vocal folds. The pressure that is built up is called subglottal pressure. Air molecules accumulate under the vocal folds until the subglottal pressure exceeds the pressure of vocal fold closure, displacing the vocal folds laterally. The vocal folds are first displaced at their bottom edge, and then at their top edge. This *vertical phase difference* is referred to as the *mucosal wave*. The air that has moved through the glottis continues its ascent through the pharynx and finally exits the body either through the mouth or nose. At the same time, the vocal folds demonstrate the same elastic tendency as the lungs. That is, after they are displaced laterally, they demonstrate a tendency to return to their original position. They close first at their bottom edge, and then at their top edge. When they are sufficiently close, the air that rushes past them tends to create a negative pressure and helps to suck them together—or at least fails to generate enough of a positive pressure to impede the process of closure. Once the bottom edge of the vocal folds completely closes, subglottal pressure builds up again and the vibratory cycle repeats (Figure A-6).

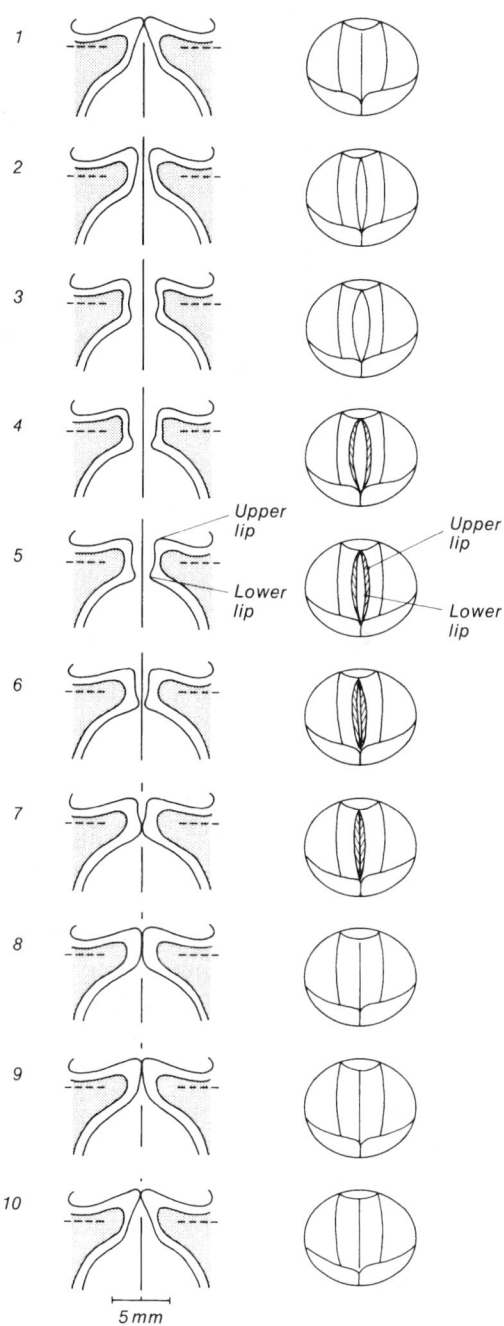

Figure A-6. A complete vibratory cycle. From *Clinical Examination of Voice*, by M. Hirano, 1981, New York: Springer-Verlag. Copyright 1981 by Springer-Verlag. With kind permission of Springer Science+Business Media.

Voicing is the result of multiple cycles of vocal fold vibration. The fundamental frequency of a voice is the number of cycles per second that the vocal folds vibrate. The average speaking *fundamental frequency* (the number of times that the vocal folds open and close each second) of a man in speech is around 110 cycles per second and a woman's is around 200 cycles per second (Baken, 1987). The psychoacoustic correlate of fundamental frequency is known as pitch, and pitch is determined by several factors including fundamental frequency and intensity. It should be noted that the voice undergoes age-related changes in response to the body's maturation. As such, the voice of a man will increase in fundamental frequency with age, whereas a woman's voice actually lowers with age. Other changes may include differences in voice quality and vocal control.

Factors Affecting Vocal Function

Of concern to directors and actors alike is whether the voice will hold up during long, demanding performance schedules. The implication of a rigorous performance schedule is that, as with the extraordinary use of other tissues in the body, repetitive and athletic use may stress the tissue, and thus will affect performance. Accordingly, in order for the actor to deliver a high-caliber performance for the duration of a theatrical run, he wants to use the voice in ways that minimize the risk of vocal injury. Two factors appear to be the most important ones in causing injury. The first factor is *phonotrauma* (Verdolini, 1999), the term used to describe change in biological tissue properties as a consequence of phonation. It is believed that the most direct causal factor for phonotrauma is vocal fold impact stress (Titze, 1994), that is, perpendicular impact stress between the vibrating vocal folds. In turn, vocal fold impact stress appears to increase with:

1. an increase in subglottic pressure (Jiang & Titze, 1994),
2. hyperadduction of the vocal folds (Berry et al., 2001; Jiang & Titze, 1994) (a configuration of the vocal folds where the vocal folds are pressed together *past* the point of barely touching, so that they are in fact overclosed), and

3. vocal fold elongation within chest register in particular (Jiang & Titze, 1994).

The second broad factor influencing vocal fold injury is inflammation of the tissue due to other (nonphonatory) causes. Primary among them are laryngopharyngeal reflux (LPR) (Koufman, 1991; Shaw & Searl, 1997; Shaw, Searl, Young, & Miner, 1996) and exposure to smoke, pollutants, subject-specific allergens, and various medications.

The next section will address several "technical" parameters that affect voice production including type of breathing, phonation mode, and variations in resonance. The Appendix will conclude with recommendations about how to care for the voice by focusing on hydration, voice use and rest schedules, and medical and environmental factors.

Breathing Issues

Several different schools of breathing technique for phonation can be identified. Two broad categories are "up and in" versus "down and out" approaches, though approaches to respiration evolve as voice trainers and scientists gain increased understanding of what is most effective. There is controversy over which approach is the "ideal" one. Some thought suggests that the ideal approach varies from actor to actor based on personal physical characteristics (Thomasson & Sundberg, 1999, 2001). As discussed shortly, there is also increasing evidence that the voice production system is highly interactive, such that the ideal approach to breathing (however ideal is defined) may depend on laryngeal and vocal tract behaviors. Therefore, when working with actors, a director should recognize that training approaches may vary (see Chapter 2, Overview of Voice Methods, Chapter 3, Overview of Speech Methods, and Chapter 4, Voice and the Alexander Technique). Interestingly, instructing a trained performer to use a different breathing process than the one in which he is trained or uses natively *may* actually interfere with voice production (Schmidt & Lee, 2005), unless the actor is in a situation where there is ample time to integrate the new technique over several months. This will sometimes occur in a situation such as the Stratford Shakespearean Festival in Canada or the Royal

Shakespeare Company, in England, where the actors have the opportunity to work with voice/dialect and Alexander coaches to integrate new habits into performance. Asking an actor to change habits in a short time requires the expert guidance of a trained coach; otherwise, it may have a less desirable outcome, one that does not accomplish the director's goal. A better approach might be to inform the actor about the desired dramatic effects and how to align his intentions in the scene to the desired effect (see Chapter 7, Voice and Text Explorations) rather than giving explicit biomechanical instructions on how to breathe—or how to produce voice mechanically, more generally.

We now proceed with the discussion of breathing in acting by considering special issues. In this venue, those issues include questions of nasal versus oral breathing, tracheal pull, and approaches to inhalation and exhalation.

Nasal Breathing versus Oral Breathing

For voice production purposes, nasal breathing is generally preferred over oral breathing for several reasons. When air enters the nose, the air is warmed, humidified, and filtered as it passes through the airway to the vocal folds. Surface desiccation of the vocal fold may result from continuous oral breathing. This effect may be heightened in many theaters in which the stage environment may be dry (Richter, Lohle, Maier, Kliemann, & Verdolini, 2000). When the vocal folds are dry, the lung pressure required to vibrate them is increased, and thus general vocal effort increases, especially at high pitches (Sivasankar & Fisher, 2002). A second possible effect of dry vocal folds is that they may be more susceptible to injury from voice use than moist folds (Titze, 1981; Verdolini-Marston, Sandage, & Titze, 1994).

That said, most of the time it is necessary for an actor to inhale through the mouth. This situation may arise because there is not enough time to take a breath through the nose due to the pacing of lines. As the nasal passages are smaller than the oral cavity, they offer more resistance to the flow of air than the mouth. The decreased rate at which air can be inhaled nasally requires the actor to take more time during inhalation, and pacing may be disrupted. In addition, the actor may make a character choice to breathe through the mouth. If, for instance, the character is supposed to be congested, the actor may elect to breathe orally instead of nasally to portray the condition of the character. Particularly in such cases and also as an adjunct to nasal breathing, backstage steam inhalers for use between entrances and during intermissions may be especially useful to help preserve the actor's ease in phonation (Jiang, Verdolini, Aquino, Ng, & Hanson, 2000; Verdolini, Titze, & Druker, 1990; Verdolini, Titze, & Fennell, 1994) and mucosal health (Verdolini-Marston et al., 1994). During intermission the actor may use the inhalers to rehydrate the vocal fold mucosa that was desiccated during the performance.

The Tracheal Pull

A positive consequence of contracting the diaphragm fully so that it has a large descent (displacing the abdominal contents outward) is that the larynx is pulled downward as a result (Iwarsson & Sundberg, 1998). That is, when the diaphragm contracts and lowers, it exerts a pull on the ribcage and lungs above it. The lungs are connected to the trachea, so if the lungs lower during diaphragmatic contraction, then the trachea should also lower. Because the larynx sits on the first ring of the trachea, it also is pulled down when the diaphragm descends. When the larynx is pulled down during this process, the vocal folds are slightly abducted (Iwarsson, Thomasson, & Sundberg, 1998). The implication is that *laryngeal* behavior varies according to how the actor breathes. Adequate diaphragmatic lowering—without forcing—may help to counteract an actor's tendencies to hyperadduct the vocal folds, thereby helping to decrease the risk of injury to them.

Inhalation during Speech Is Quick and Imperceptible

Inhalation is usually accomplished quickly during speech. The short duration of inhalation allows a person to speak with minimal disruption to the flow of speech. Changes in lung compliance (i.e., the ability of the tissue to stretch) can cause problems with inhalation. Certain conditions change the compliance of lung tissue, such as conditions arising from smoking. When the tissue is less compliant, increases in lung volume during inhalation are impaired. As a result, the actor may require more time to inhale, and, consequently, interrupt the delivery of lines. The fragmentation of lines may lead

to disastrous dramatic effects because
ate build of ideas of the scene and, hen   ……ural flow
of the scene and the production.

Additionally, because of various lung conditions due to smoking and other causes, the actor may not be able to inhale an adequate amount of air for the communication of given thoughts. When the volume of available inhaled air is decreased, the actor's speech patterns may need to be altered. The actor may need to take more frequent breaths when speaking. If the actor tries to speak beyond the volume of air that is inhaled, the actor may attempt to squeeze more air out to finish the utterance, which has been shown to involve hyperadduction of the vocal folds and potential injury. Specifically, the vocal folds adduct as an attempt to help slow down the outflow of air at low lung volumes, and the result is a "pressed" sounding voice, the biomechanical correlate of which may be harmful to the tissue and, moreover, may compromise the expression of thoughts.

Another issue has to do with sounds associated with inhalation. The process of inhalation should be imperceptible. Sometimes, an actor may have a "noisy breath" during inhalation. This is particularly problematic when the actor is using a microphone, as the noise will be amplified. The same effect occurs in film or any electronic media where microphones are used (see Chapter 9, Special Issues, Use of Microphones). This result could be due to vocal fold approximation during inhalation, which not only counteracts the inspiratory effort, but also may increase the tendency for the vocal folds to press together during subsequent voicing. Most voice and speech trainers would agree that the preferred manner of inhalation involves minimal, if any, audible noise because the larynx has to be relatively relaxed and the vocal folds wide open to accomplish this end.

Musculoskeletal tension patterns and alignment may also affect inhalation. For instance, an actor who holds the muscles of the abdomen tight will restrict how much the diaphragm lowers by impeding the down and outward displacement of the abdominal contents—a typical consequence of diaphragmatic contraction and lowering. Likewise, an actor who uses a hunched body position while standing may limit the ribcage's mobility and ability to expand and contract. Both of these issues may result in limiting the amount of air that can be inhaled. Of course, standing with a hunched posture may be required if an actor is portraying an older character, for example, and speaking the lines in shorter phrases would reflect the impact of that type of physicality on a person's speech. That said, it is important in such an instance to find the more easeful way to achieve the physicality of the character (see Chapter 4, Voice and the Alexander Technique).

Exhalation during Speech Is Usually Slow and Controlled

Because an egressive airstream (in which airflow is in the direction of inside to outside the body) is required to vibrate the vocal folds during normal speech, clearly exhalation, or what Kristin Linklater refers to as the "release of breath," is key to the production of voice. For humans, after the onset of speech, exhalation is typically extended longer than inhalation during both rest breathing and speech. The actor needs to release air judiciously in order to be able to complete most utterances, which is why the actor needs to understand the specifics of the thought process. His overall vocal mechanism can respond to the specific needs of the text with the appropriate amount of release time on the exhalation. During exhalation, various muscles control how much air is released. First, when air is expelled from the lungs during phonation, the opening and closing of the vocal folds alters the flow of air and, as a result, typically reduces the amount of air that flows into the atmosphere, compared to the amount during breathing at rest.

In addition, the muscles of exhalation and inhalation control how much air is released at any given moment. Think of a balloon. If you choose to release the air from a balloon that is inflated, the air can be released quickly by letting the neck of the balloon open completely, or it can be released slowly by pinching the neck of the balloon. By narrowing the neck of the balloon, the airflow is reduced and it takes longer for all of the air to be released. The same principle is true for phonation: good vocal fold closure, along with simultaneous activation of *inspiratory* muscles during exhalation (paradoxically, attempting to *expand* the ribcage and lungs during exhalation), will help to limit the amount of air that flows out of the lungs for any given unit of time. Thus, the air will last longer. However, overclosure of the vocal folds as occurs for pressed voice will not necessarily preserve air any better than "barely touching" vocal folds, and the risk of vocal fold injury increases (Berry et al., 2001; Jiang & Titze, 1994). Therefore, especially for long utterances, inspiratory gestures should be made at the same time as expiratory gestures to slow the airflow and avoid vocal fold pressing. During speech, which has been previously described as an action that takes place during exhalation, the actor should offset the muscular forces that push the air out of the lungs by continuing to engage the inspiratory muscles, especially where long phrases are concerned. By having these two opposing muscle groups—inspiratory and exhalatory—engaged simultaneously, the air can be sustained for a greater duration. On a practical level, keep the ribcage expanded as you speak long phrases.

The respiratory muscles are not only important regulators of airflow through the glottis; they also contribute to vocal loudness by adjusting subglottal pressure, which is similar to the pressure in the lungs. If all other factors are held constant, increases in subglottal pressure increase voice output intensity, which is related to loudness (loudness being the psychoacoustic correlate of intensity). The actor may increase subglottal (and lung) pressure by (a) contracting the abdominal muscles and displacing the abdominal wall in, an action that pushes the diaphragm up and reduces lung volume, and/or (b) reducing the ribcage dimensions during phonation. In some approaches, the reduction of the ribcage is delayed on phonation (i.e., the ribs are held out for a longer time as the actor is speaking, to increase the potential length of the phrase and/or loudness). The latter example is what some trainers mean by *support*—although the exact meaning in physiological terms may vary greatly across trainers. As a person increases subglottal pressure to generate greater vocal intensity, the amplitude of vocal fold vibration also increases. In other words, the excursion from midline to the point of maximal separation that the vocal folds travel is greater. Conversely, less subglottal pressure creates smaller amplitude vocal fold vibrations. A consequence of increasing subglottal pressure by generating larger lung pressure values is that there may also be an increase in the amount and rate of airflow through the glottis. This situation results in a relatively rapid depletion of air in the lungs. As more air is being used during any given interval of time, the actor will generally have less time available to speak on one breath. This factor can be counterbalanced, as discussed above, by increasing work in the *inspiratory* muscles during phonation, to help slow down the airflow. However, a caution is that an increase in subglottic pressure also leads to an increase in the impact stress between the vocal folds, if all other factors are held constant (Jiang & Titze, 1994). As a result, large subglottal pressures —sometimes generated as the result of what some trainers consider support—could inadvertently contribute to phonotrauma. This is why it is important that actors be guided through these issues by expert voice trainers who are familiar with ways to minimize tension that could potentially increase the risk of phonotrauma.

Phonation Issues

Voice Quality and Vocal Strain

Pressed voice and breathy voice represent extremes in a continuum of how the vocal folds are postured during voice production. A pressed voice is considered to be hyperfunctional, or "strained," overfunctioning because the manner of production involves a literal pressing of the vocal folds together, with considerable compression and force. In pressed voice, the closed phase of each vocal fold vibratory cycle is longer in duration than the open phase. On the other hand, a breathy voice involves vocal folds that are fairly far apart during phonation, at least at some point along their length. As a result, a substantial amount of air may escape through the glottis without being turned into systematic sound waves (voice). Due to limited activation of laryngeal muscles, this type of voice production may be hypofunctional (an abnormal, minimal amount of activity, or underuse). However, in some cases, breathy voice can be associated with simultaneous contraction of both the vocal fold adductor and abductor muscles at the same time. Indeed, most directors have heard strained, breathy voices, which often are associated with this sort of pattern. In some cases, pressed or breathy voice may be an actor or director's choice. In other cases, the cause is simply bad technique that may be harmful to the effective voice production. Moreover, vocal loudness is generally decreased with either pressed or breathy voice. Although such voice qualities may be useful for certain character portrayals, directors should be mindful that both pressed and strained, breathy voice as the *base* voice for the character may put the actor at risk for fatigue, if not injury, during the course of a show.

Whispering

During breathy voice production, the vocal folds continue to vibrate and create some degree of systematic sound waves. However, during a whisper, the vocal folds do not vibrate at all. A whisper results from keeping the vocal folds tensed but generally abducted (although in some cases the folds actually touch during whispering). Air rushes through the glottis, causing frication. The audible noise that is produced is what the listener hears. There is controversy about whether or not whispering can be harmful to the vocal folds. It is likely that certain types of "tense" whisper may be harmful, as the vocal folds can indeed touch during a whisper, even though they do not vibrate. Moreover, aerodynamic features of high-pressure frication are potentially harmful; but it is likely that an "easy whisper" is not harmful. However, an easy whisper is almost impossible to hear from the stage without extremely competent articulation, and is rarely used on stage. The term *stage whisper* is often used when directing actors, especially in an aside to the audience as is often seen in Shakespeare. The ideal stage whisper consists of the previously mentioned easy whisper together with the use of precise and even crisp articulation.

Vocal Considerations for Character Choices

Character voices and screaming or yelling on stage are important vocal demands to address. As a rule of thumb, producing voice in a manner that causes hyperfunction of the laryngeal mechanism should never be encouraged. In addition to pressing (or tense abduction) of the vocal folds, hyperfunction may involve a squeezing together of the false vocal folds (paired folds located superior to the true vocal folds that consist of thick muscular tissue), resulting in a narrowed supraglottic space. The narrowed space is not, of itself, a concern, and various approaches to singing pedagogy in particular have indicated such narrowed space may be an important source of the "ring" that is heard in good classical singing and acting voices. However, extreme pressing that may occur with onstage screaming and yelling may be harmful. There are ways to achieve the target effects that do not require hyperfunction. For example, the actor can explore manipulating resonance (see Chapter 6, Resonex). Another attractive option is for the actor to receive specialized training in screaming, with a qualified vocal coach, to minimize the risk of injury.

Other vocal behaviors required for the portrayal of a character may similarly demand certain behaviors that could be harmful to vocal fold tissue. Coughing and throat clearing are two examples. Both of these behaviors cause the vocal folds to adduct in a relatively forceful manner and potentially induce large intrafold stresses. Every time an actor coughs and clears the throat, the vocal folds may be subject to a great amount of impact stress, particularly if these behaviors are aggressive. As already noted, impact stress in turn can generate phonotrauma, and, therefore, it may be important to limit the amount of forceful coughing and throat-clearing an actor is required to perform. If these behaviors are required in a production, it is best to limit and especially space out their use in rehearsals and performance.

Vocal Fold Injury Due to Phonation

One of directors' and actors' primary concerns has to do with vocal fold injury. As with athletes who have demanding performance schedules, actors are also susceptible to injury in the parts of the body required for the job. Due to the inherent structure of the vocal fold, the mucosa is particularly susceptible to phonotrauma or injury due to voice use. As the outermost portion of the vocal fold, the mucosa of one vocal fold contacts the mucosa of the other fold 100 to 1,000 times per second during phonation. Over the course of the day, the number of vocal fold collisions may be 1,000,000 or greater, depending on the amount and pitch of voice use. Each time the vocal folds collide, they are subjected to mechanical stress. The situation is further compounded by the amount of force with which the vocal folds collide. As the vocal folds return to midline they accelerate, generating a force upon impact. As already noted, that force—or stress (force per unit area)—is increased by vocal fold lengthening (increased pitch) at least in chest voice, by increased subglottal pressure, and by pressing the vocal folds together. Stated differently, vocal fold impact stress tends to increase with increasing pitch, increasing loudness, and especially increased pressing of the vocal folds. If the impact stress to the tissue exceeds certain thresholds over time, the risk of injury increases, probably partly depending on the individual's personal biological profile. Injury from phonation can manifest as many different clinical entities ranging from inflammation and edema (swelling) to frank lesions such as nodules, polyps, vocal fold scar, or fibrous mass, and possibly cysts and sulcus vocalis; the last involves a groove in the vocal fold tissue. Physical changes associated with such injuries tend to alter the mucosa's vibratory pattern, and, as a result, there is a change in vocal fold function. Over the past few decades, considerable knowledge has been gained about the biological profile associated with phonotraumatic injury. Treatment options have increased, and such injury is no longer necessarily the kiss of professional death that it was in the past. However, it is clear that avoidance of injury remains the operative goal for actors.

Signs of Hyperfunction

Two types of vocal hyperfunction have been identified. One of them involves *hyper*adduction, which we have already cited as a cardinal cause of injury to the vocal fold tissue. The other type actually involves *hypo*adduction, the cocontraction of opposing muscle groups in the larynx such that the *ab*ductor muscles keep the *ad*ductor muscles from accomplishing their task of bringing the vocal folds together. Hyperadduction can lead to vocal fold injury. Hypoadduction does not usually cause injury in the vocal folds, but can cause a sense of extremely effortful voicing.

Hyperfunction of either type in an actor can arise as an attempt to create a desired effect. For instance, if an actor wants to increase loudness, he has three options. The first is to increase subglottic pressure. The second is to increase vocal fold adduction (but not to the point of pressing the vocal folds together, which paradoxically actually *decreases* vocal loudness). The third is to "tune" the vocal tract to the frequencies produced by the vocal folds, to maximally amplify them. Tuning is the approach that is least costly to the tissue, and is implicitly taught by many voice and speech coaches who teach adjustment of the oral and pharyngeal cavities to manipulate sound. An increase in vocal fold adduction—to a point—can be a relatively safe approach to increasing loudness. However, many actors go beyond the threshold for "safe" adduction and press their vocal folds together to increase loudness. In that case, they are not only actually *decreasing* their loudness but, as noted, they are also simultaneously increasing their risk of injury. Increasing subglottal pressure also increases the risk of injury, and may need to be offset by decreased vocal fold adduction and/or vocal tract tuning.

One question that is often asked is whether vocal hyperfunction of either type can be deduced by visible contraction of the neck muscles and prominence of blood vessels in the neck. Although this conclusion makes sense intuitively, in fact, there is little evidence that such observations are clear indicators of hyperfunction—otherwise known as "bad vocal technique." One need only think of selected premier singers in whom these manifestations are common. Potentially, some individuals have less fatty tissue in the neck than others, and blood vessels are simply more visually prominent when an actor increases subglottal pressure—itself not a negative event in limited doses—and thus blood flow through the neck increases. In sum, the sense of the actor's overall physical *effort* may be a greater indicator of hyperfunction than any visual cues in the neck.

In contrast, evidence of jaw "gripping" (heightened contraction of the jaw muscles) may be a more reliable indicator of vocal hyperfunction. The mandible attaches to the larynx through a muscular connection to the hyoid bone. Moreover, neurological connections exist between jaw and laryngeal innervations. Some evidence suggests that these latter connections may be avenues through which tight jaw muscles may reflect, or even cause, laryngeal hyperfunction that is both esthetically limiting and potentially harmful to the tissue. The tongue can be another source of tension that results in voice problems. (See Chapter 5, Vox Explora.) Like the jaw, the tongue is connected to the larynx through a muscular attachment to the hyoid bone. One generally assumes that tongue tension can cause the larynx to rise up in the pharynx and limit the larynx from moving freely.

Being Heard and Understood: Filling a Space or Projection

A goal of the director is for the actor to be heard. If the actor simply attempts to get "louder," the result is often a pressed voice. As noted, this voicing type appears to increase the risk of injury to the tissue compared to other voicing types, due to an increase in vocal fold impact stress. Moreover, pressing actually *decreases* loudness, so the actor's attempts will be foiled *and* he may become injured (Berry et al., 2001). The actor may also change the resonance to increase loudness. (See Chapter 6, Resonex.) When the actor changes the size and shape of the vocal tract, certain frequencies become amplified. *Mask resonance* is a type of resonance that involves a prominence of vibrations on the septum of the nose, the zygomatic arch, the lips, and the alveolar ridge. Voice produced with this resonance often carries well in a large theater. In the final analysis, however, if the actor is properly trained and has a healthy vocal mechanism, and if he commits fully to communicating his objective with precise yet easeful articulation and the intent to include those in the last row, generally he will be heard.

Environmental Acoustics

Once the actor is inside the space in which a performance is to take place, the space should be tested for its acoustics. The director should have the actor speak, and then listen for the reverberation as it bounces off the back wall. If the voice does not produce an echo, the actor should experiment with making necessary adjustments in subglottal pressure, resonance, and/or articulation to achieve an echo. In some cases, the actor attempts to produce more voice than is actually required to fill the space. However, the acoustics in some spaces are such that the voice does not carry well regardless of the approach. These are called acoustically dead spaces. No matter what the actor does, the vocal signal will not reach the back of the audience in a satisfying way. In this type of space, the actor should not be encouraged to try to project more than is healthy. If, after adjustments are made, voice modulations still do not reach the last row of the space in a way that can be readily perceived, then other arrangements should be made for the actor to be heard. A few options include the use of microphones to help amplify the voice (see Chapter 9, Special Issues, Use of Microphones) or an alteration in the staging so that the actors are positioned closer to the audience for critical lines.

Nonphonatory Tissue Care

Hormonal Influence

Phonation is affected by life events such as puberty, the menstrual cycle, and menopause that vary sex hormone levels and result in changes to the larynx. Such effects are partly due to receptors located in the larynx that respond to fluctuations in hormones (Amir & Biron-Shental, 2004). During puberty, sex hormones such as androgens cause laryngeal cartilage to grow larger and the vocal folds to become bulkier. As a result of the change in anatomy, the fundamental frequency in both males and females lowers, but males experience a more dramatic voice change than females. After puberty, the male voice remains relatively stable. On the other hand, the female voice is subject to other hormonal processes that affect the voice throughout the lifespan.

Every month the female body undergoes hormonal changes associated with a process known as menstruation. Voice disturbances that occur from changes in hormone levels immediately preceding menstruation are called *laryngopathia premenstrualis* and consist of mild hoarseness, diminished voice range, vocal inefficiency, and vocal fatigue. Dysphonia similar to laryngopathia premenstrualis is also seen during the ovulatory phase of the menstrual cycle. In addition to voice changes, cramping during menstruation may impair the actor's ability to effectively use abdominal muscles during phonation. Some females take oral contraceptives to regulate hormone levels and minimize symptoms from menstruation (Amir & Kishon-Rabin, 2004; Amir, Kishon-Rabin, & Muchnik, 2002), but there is concern that some (but not all) forms of this medication may cause voice changes. In the United States, progesterone levels in oral contraceptives are low enough that there is little risk of masculinizing the voice.

The female body decreases production of estrogen during menopause and eventually loses the capability of reproducing. This process results in further voice changes. Singers both undergoing and already completing menopause commonly complain of voice disturbances such as pitch breaks, breathiness, loss of high pitches, change in timbre, and decreased vocal flexibility. After menopause, females continue to produce androgens and, as a result, the voice lowers permanently. Hormone replacement therapy, in which females take estrogen, delays the effects of menopause on voice production.

Hormonal disturbances due to endocrine dysfunction such as thyroid and pituitary gland tumors may also result in temporary and permanent voice disruption. Consequently, consultation among the endocrinologist, gynecologist (for female actors), and otolaryngologist is necessary for effective medical management that minimizes risk to the actor's voice. The actor should be made aware of the risks to the voice from treatment before the course of treatment begins.

Hydration

The larynx is definitely a resilient structure, but how it is cared for is crucial for its health and optimum voicing results. Returning to the issue of hydration, first, adequate systemic and surface (ambient) hydration appears important for normal voice production. Diuretics such as caffeine increase water removal from the body, systemically. Similarly, dry environments, mouth breathing, and certain drugs (e.g., antihistamines, decongestants, and selected psychotropic drugs) can dehydrate the vocal folds superficially. In both cases, two negative effects may occur. First, the subglottic pressure required for phonation may increase (Fisher, Ligon, Sobecks, & Roxe, 2001; Jiang et al., 2000; Titze, 1988; Verdolini et al., 2002; Verdolini et al., 1990; Verdolini et al., 1994)—especially at high pitches—making phonation physically more taxing for the actor. Second, the risk of injury to the tissue with phonation may increase (Titze, 1981). Clearly, adequate systemic and surface hydration is needed to optimize vocal fold structure and function. An interesting note is that at least with respect to subglottic pressure, deleterious effects of systemic dehydration may first be seen *several hours* after the dehydrating event. In practical terms, if an actor has to decide whether to work out (and hence perspire) in the morning before an evening show or a few hours before the show, from the perspective of vocal fold hydration, a few hours closer to the performance may be best. In any case, good systemic rehydration will be required to optimize function.

Environmental Factors

As noted, the vocal fold epithelium is a barrier that protects the internal environment of the body from foreign substances. Only certain particles are able to pass through the cells that line the vocal tract and the rest of the airway, thereby limiting unwanted particles from disrupting the activity of the internal environment. If one considers the "environment" as any element originating outside the larynx itself, one environmental condition that may affect voice is laryngopharyngeal reflux, or LPR (Koufman, 1991; Shaw & Searl, 1997; Shaw et al., 1996). LPR is a medical condition characterized by the regurgitation of gastric juices that spill over into the larynx and irritate the mucosa. The tissue usually becomes inflamed. Medication for LPR may reduce reflux or at least reflux's acidity, but those who are troubled by this condition are also usually advised to make dietary and other behavioral changes, such as losing weight (if relevant), avoidance of exercise or sleep for a few hours after eating, and possibly sleeping with an elevated head.

Other environmental factors that may affect the actor's voice in particular are factors inherent to the theater environment itself. Empirical research has revealed that stage environments can host an astounding array of chemicals, dust, mildew, and other elements that have definite potential to negatively affect the actor's vocal folds (Richter et al., 2002; Richter et al., 2000). Harmful chemicals on stage include, but are not limited to, those that come from paints, fog machines, and cigarette smoking. Dust and mildew are as much a part of theaters, especially older theaters, as are the actors. All of these substances can affect the epithelial cells in the upper and lower airway. The body has sensory receptors located throughout the airway that react to irritants such as chemicals and dust. One effect may be an inflammatory response that limits vocal fold mucosal function and, moreover, may become progressive. These irritants may also trigger a coughing response that not only harms the tissue, but also harms the show. The director should take measures to minimize the irritants with which the actor will come into contact. It is recommended that the director use fog solutions and paints that limit harm. (See Use of Fog or Smoke, or Presence of Dust in the Theater in Chapter 9, Special Issues.) Consultation with a pharmacist or biologist may be in order, and, in some cases, investigation of the concentrations of harmful substances on stage may be warranted so that appropriate actions may be taken. Also, it may be helpful for the stage and set to be thoroughly cleaned regularly to minimize the amount of dust particles that result from set construction. Prolonged exposure to such irritants may disrupt normal function of the vocal mechanism such that the actor is unable to perform to the necessary level.

Voice Use and Voice Rest

Priming the Voice with a Warm-Up

Voice and speech trainers agree that a vocal warm-up is useful, if not essential, for helping the actor meet the demands of a performance. (See Chapter 5, Vox Explora.) The general thought is that a thorough warm-up can prime the voice biologically and biomechanically, literally increasing the temperature of the muscles. It also focuses the attention of the actor. Imagine driving a car on a cold winter morning without letting it warm up. The car functions, but it does not accelerate easily. It is sluggish. The voice appears to be similar in many cases. There is some thought that the warm-up serves to "loosen up" the muscles. Specifically, as for other skeletal muscles, a warm-up should increase blood flow to the muscles involved. Such flow provides them with more oxygen, which is required for the contraction of "endurance" muscles, which characterize essential portions of the intrinsic laryngeal musculature. Also, when engaged in a warm-up, the actor becomes aware of the breathing pattern employed and perceives vibrations produced by the acoustic waves emanating from the vocal folds in different regions such as the face. The actor needs to learn to monitor voice use. This kinesthetic feedback is important for just that reason. The sensations that accompany voice production heighten the actor's perception of the voice that is being produced. The corollary is that evidence also suggests that the perception of vibrations in the front of the face, together with a sense that voice is "easy," is an indicator that the vocal folds are getting together sufficiently to make a rich, brilliant sound but are not pressing in a way that is harmful to the tissue (Verdolini, 2000; Verdolini-Marston, Burke, Lessac, Glaze, & Caldwell, 1995).

Voice Conservation, Cool-Down, and Rest

The muscles used in voice production, like other muscles in the body, are subject to both fatigue and injury. Fatigue occurs when muscles are not able to sustain a certain level of activity. Interestingly, not only vocal muscles but also vocal fold mucosa can demonstrate "fatigue," understood as failure to perform at consistent levels over time, subsequent to use of the tissue. As already discussed, injury can also ensue with certain kinds of tissue use. Actors need to be aware of personal thresholds for vocal fatigue and injury, and pace voice use accordingly. Voice conservation is one approach to limiting fatigue and injury. Conservation does not mean that the actor does not use the voice, but instead uses the voice in moderation. For instance, during rehearsals, instead of always speaking lines at performance level, the actor may choose to speak the lines at a less intense level. This technique is called *marking*, a term also used in the dance world for walking through a choreographic sequence without full physical commitment. The director and other actors should be aware when actors are marking, in order to adjust expectations accordingly. Whispering is not a good substitution for marking.

Another important issue has to do most directly with vocal fold injury that occurs to some degree—albeit usually subclinically—in most individuals on a daily basis. For the actor, who may experience greater levels of injury, one interesting approach that has recently received attention in the voice science community has to do with voice "cool-downs." Cool-downs have been advocated by a number of practitioners for some time. However, recent data from the basic science community indicates that cool-downs in the form of *resonant voice exercises* (e.g., humming easily, with strong vibrations in the front of the mouth) may actually assist with the reduction of vocal fold inflammation, *in some cases more than voice rest*. More specifically, a cool-down routine generally consists of engaging the actor in light voice exercises that "feel good"—especially those with vibrations in the front of the face—for a period of several minutes, up to 10 to 20 minutes on and off. (Also see Chapter 5, Vox Explora.)

Voice rest, or a period of nonvoicing, is another strategy that is vitally important for maintaining normal vocal function as well. The thought is that the tissue can withstand and recover from traumatic forces better if a given amount of phonation is distributed over time—interspersed with silence—than if it is concentrated in time, allowing for rest after the fact. Accordingly, rehearsal should never be nonstop for a given actor. (See Chapter 8, Directors, Voice, and the Rehearsal Process.) The actor should be given time to rest the voice during rehearsal. One suggestion is to block scenes without requiring the actors to speak their lines. Once the scene is blocked, the rehearsal of the scene can incorporate speaking lines. If the goal of the rehearsal is just to review the staging, then the actor might be encouraged to mark his lines. Another way to provide the actor with voice rest is by staggering scenes. For instance, rehearse one scene in which the actor is involved and then block a scene in which the actor is not needed. Not allowing sufficient recovery time for the voice between periods of intense use on or off stage may have detrimental effects to the tissue's structure and function.

We now turn to the issue of sleep. There never seems to be enough time to prepare an actor in a production for performance. The week before a production opens can be exhausting. Sleep may benefit the actor in several ways. First, while sleeping, the vocal folds are basically abducted and largely inactive. As a result of tissue rest, together with the reparative biological properties associated with sleep in general, the vocal folds can recover from the insults to which they were subjected during the day. Second, sleep is necessary for recharging the body and mind. After a night's rest, the actor will have the physical energy of the rest of the body to support the production of voice and perform. In addition, by refueling not just the body but also the mind, the actor will have greater focus and be able to monitor behaviors such as voice use. Finally, sleep is important to consolidate new learned behavior.

Pain . . . No Gain

Finally, voice production *should never* involve pain. Pain is a sign that the manner of voice production is not healthy. A director should take an actor's complaint of pain or discomfort while voicing extremely seriously and take necessary steps to help the actor prevent further vocal difficulties. Alternatives for achieving what is being required vocally should be explored. Unhealthy production can lead to temporary or even permanent damage to the voice.

Concluding Remarks

The actor's vocal well-being should be of utmost concern for the director. The slightest deviation from normal voice production, if left untreated, can have devastating effects on a theatrical production, including absences from rehearsal and performances. An actor may feel ashamed or fear that his role is at stake if it is known that there is difficulty with voice production. As discussed previously, voice problems may be due to one or multiple etiologies, and the way in which an actor produces voice is just one possible contributing factor. Indicators of damage to the voice suggest early intervention, rather than later. The director, with proper awareness and education, can support healthy voice usage by taking advantage of the talents and expertise of voice/speech trainers, Alexander coaches, and the interdisciplinary network of laryngologists and speech-language pathologists dedicated to caring for the professional voice user. Collaborating with the voice/speech coach, the laryngologist and the speech-language pathologist, and referring appropriately—again sooner rather than later—can make the difference between a vocally dynamic performance contributing to the success of a production and a distracting vocal performance that may end up causing huge inconveniences to the overall production.

REFERENCES

Amir, O., & Biron-Shental, T. (2004). The impact of hormonal fluctuations on female vocal folds. *Current Opinions in Otolaryngology–Head and Neck Surgery*, *12*(3), 180–184.

Amir, O., & Kishon-Rabin, L. (2004). Association between birth control pills and voice quality. *Laryngoscope*, *114*(6), 1021–1026.

Amir, O., Kishon-Rabin, L., & Muchnik, C. (2002). The effect of oral contraceptives on voice: Preliminary observations. *Journal of Voice*, *16*(2), 267–273.

Ardran, G. M., & Kemp, F. H. (1956). Closure and opening of the larynx during swallowing. *British Journal of Radiology*, *29*(340), 205–208.

Baken, R. J. (1987). *Clinical measurement of voice and speech*. Boston: College Hill Press.

Berry, D. A., Verdolini, K., Montequin, D., Hess, M. M., Chan, R., &, Titze, I. R. (2001). A quantitative output-cost ratio in voice production. *Journal of Speech, Language, and Hearing Research*, *44*(1), 29–37.

Bryant, N. J., Woodson, G. E., Kaufman, K., Rosen, C., Hengesteg, A., Chen, N., et al. (1996). Human posterior cricoarytenoid muscle compartments. Anatomy and mechanics. *Archives of Otolaryngology–Head Neck Surgery*, *122*(12), 1331–1336.

Fisher, K. V., Ligon, J., Sobecks, J. L., & Roxe, D. M. (2001). Phonatory effects of body fluid removal. *Journal of Speech, Language, and Hearing Research*, *44*, 354–367.

Gray, S. D., Pignatari, S. S., & Harding, P. (1994). Morphologic ultrastructure of anchoring fibers in normal vocal fold basement membrane zone. *Journal of Voice*, *8*(1), 48–52.

Hammond, T. H., Gray, S. D., & Butler, J. E. (2000). Age- and gender-related collagen distribution in human vocal folds. *Annals of Otology, Rhinology, and Laryngology, 109*(10 Pt. 1), 913-920.

Hammond, T. H., Gray, S. D., Butler, J., Zhou, R., & Hammond, E. (1998). A study of age and gender related elastin distribution changes in human vocal folds. *Otolaryngology-Head and Neck Surgery, 119*, 314-322.

Hixon, T. J., &. Jeannette, D. (2005). *Evaluation and management of speech breathing disorders: Principles and methods* (1st ed.). Tucson, AZ: Redington Brown.

Iwarsson, J., & Sundberg, J. (1998). Effects of lung volume on vertical larynx position during phonation. *Journal of Voice, 12*(2), 159-165.

Iwarsson, J., Thomasson, M., & Sundberg, J. (1998). Effects of lung volume on the glottal voice source. *Journal of Voice, 12*(4), 424-433.

Jiang, J., Verdolini, K., Aquino, B., Ng, J., & Hanson, D. (2000). Effects of dehydration on phonation in excised canine larynges. *Annals of Otology, Rhinology, and Laryngology, 109*, 568-575.

Jiang, J. J., & Titze, I. R. (1994). Measurement of vocal fold intraglottal pressure and impact stress. *Journal of Voice, 8*(2), 132-144.

Koufman, J. A. (1991). The otolaryngologic manifestations of gastroesophageal reflux disease (GERD): A clinical investigation of 225 patients using ambulatory 24-hour pH monitoring and an experimental investigation of the role of acid and pepsin in the development of laryngeal injury. *Laryngoscope, 101*(4 Pt 2 Suppl. 53), 1-78.

Richter, B., Lohle, E., Knapp, B., Weikert, M., Schlomicher-Thier, J., & Verdolini, K. (2002). Harmful substances on the opera stage: Possible negative effects on singers' respiratory tracts. *Journal of Voice, 16*(1), 72-80.

Richter, B., Lohle, E., Maier, W., Kliemann, B., & Verdolini, K. (2000). Working conditions on stage: Climatic considerations. *Logopedics, Phoniatrics, Vocology, 25*(2), 80-86.

Sataloff, R. T. (2005). *Professional voice: The science and art of clinical care* (3rd ed.). San Diego, CA: Plural.

Schmidt, R. A., & Lee, T. D. (2005). *Motor control and learning. A behavioral emphasis* (4th ed.). Champaign, IL: Human Kinetics.

Shaw, G. Y., & Searl, J. P. (1997). Laryngeal manifestations of gastroesophageal reflux before and after treatment with omeprazole. *Southern Medical Journal, 90*(11), 1115-1122.

Shaw, G. Y., Searl, J. P., Young, J. L., & Miner, P. B. (1996). Subjective, laryngoscopic, and acoustic measurements of laryngeal reflux before and after treatment with omeprazole. *Journal of Voice, 10*(4), 410-418.

Sivasankar, M., & Fisher, K. V. (2002). Oral breathing increases Pth and vocal effort by superficial drying of vocal fold mucosa. *Journal of Voice, 16*(2), 172-181.

Sundberg, J. (1977). *The acoustics of the singing voice*. New York: Scientific American.

Tateya, T., Tateya, I., & Bless, D. M. (2006). Collagen subtypes in human vocal folds. *Annals of Otology, Rhinology, and Laryngology, 115*(6), 469-476.

Thomasson, M., & Sundberg, J. (1999). Consistency of phonatory breathing patterns in professional operatic singers. *Journal of Voice, 13*(4), 529-541.

Thomasson, M., & Sundberg, J. (2001). Consistency of inhalatory breathing patterns in professional operatic singers. *Journal of Voice, 15*(3), 373-383.

Titze, I. R. (1981). Heat generation in the vocal folds and its possible effect on vocal endurance. In V. L. Lawrence (Ed.), *Transcripts of the tenth symposium: Care of the professional voice. Part 1: Instrumentation in voice research* (pp. 52-65). New York: The Voice Foundation.

Titze, I. R. (1988). The physics of small-amplitude oscillation of the vocal folds. *The Journal of the Acoustical Society of America, 83*(4), 1536-1552.

Titze, I. R. (1994). *Principles of voice production*. Englewood Cliffs, NJ: Prentice-Hall.

Verdolini, K. (1999). Critical analysis of common terminology in voice therapy: A position paper. *Phonoscope, 2*(1), 1-8.

Verdolini, K. (2000). Resonant voice therapy. In J. Stemple (Ed.), *Voice therapy: Clinical studies* (2nd ed., pp. 46-61). San Diego, CA: Singular.

Verdolini, K., Min, Y., Titze, I. R., Lemke, J., Brown, K., van Mersbergen, M., et al. (2002). Biological mechanisms underlying voice changes due to dehydration. *Journal of Speech, Language, and Hearing Research, 45*, 268-281.

Verdolini, K., Titze, I. R., & Druker, D. G. (1990). Changes in phonation threshold pressure with induced conditions of hydration. *Journal of Voice, 4*(2), 142-151.

Verdolini, K., Titze, I. R., & Fennell, A. (1994). Dependence of phonatory effort on hydration level. *Journal of Speech and Hearing Research, 37*(5), 1001-1007.

Verdolini-Marston, K., Burke, M. K., Lessac, A., Glaze, L., & Caldwell, E. (1995). Preliminary study of two methods of treatment for laryngeal nodules. *Journal of Voice, 9*(1), 74-85.

Verdolini-Marston, K., Sandage, M., & Titze, I. R. (1994). Effect of hydration treatments on laryngeal nodules and polyps and related voice measures. *Journal of Voice, 8*(1), 30-47.

Zemlin, W. (1998). *Speech and hearing science: Anatomy and physiology* (4th ed.). Boston: Allyn & Bacon.

Index

A

"Ain't I a Woman?", 67
Abraham, F. Murray, 36, 139, 182
   dialects, 34
   healthy voice usage of, 7
   and Shakespeare, 32
accent(s)
   breath support for, 145
   coaching, 142
   defined, 143
   early study of, 146
   French, 143
   German, 4
   in Shakespeare, 32
   Ybuzz resonator in, 98
Acker, Barbara, 112
acoustics
   specialists, 155
   testing, 234
acting notes
   and healthy voice usage, 133
actors
   sensitivity to, 136
   support of by coach, 176
Actors' Equity, 166
actors' resistance to voice coaching, 177
Adams, Joey Lauren
   unhealthy voice usage of, 9
Age of Innocence, The, 143
Alexander, A. R., 49
Alexander Alliance, 49, 129
   training, 49
Alexander Alliance School (Germany), 50
Alexander coach
   benefits of, 186
   responsibilities of, 187
   roles of, 186
   space to work, 187
   voice/acting background of, 187
Alexander, F. M., 45
   about, 47
Alexander Technique, 45, 57, *See* Chapter 4
   actor training in, 54
   alignment, 45
   author's experiences with, 49
   benefits for director, 51
   breath support in, 46
   chair work, 56
   conscious control, 57
   constructive rest in, 54
   development of, 46
   director training in, 54
   end gaining, 47
   and Feldenkrais, 56
   fight choreography, 54
   inhibition, 47
   and The Journey (Parks), 22
   means whereby, 47
   performance application, 48
   position of mechanical advantage or "monkey" work, 48, 56

Alexander Technique *(continued)*
  principles of, 45
  rehearsal explorations, 57
  response to text, 18
  rib reserve, 20
  speech training, 39
  table work, 56
  teacher training in, 55
  voice approach in, 43
Alice in Wonderland
  Resonex with, 90
alignment
  Alexander Technique, 45
  breath support, 45
  breathing, 226
allergies, 141
Amadeus, 7
ambient noise, minimizing, 155
American actors
  and text analysis, 19
American Conservatory Theater, San Francisco, 58
American Federation of Television and Radio Artists (AFTRA), 167
American Institute for Voice and Ear Research, 140
American Laboratory Theatre, 36
American Repertory Theatre (Harvard), 36
  and Moscow Art Theatre, 19, 21
Analyze This, 7, 8
anatomy of voice. *See* Appendix
Anderson, Claudia, 41
Ark Theatre, 40
Armstrong, Richard, 23, 89, 104
articulators
  defined, 14
ask list, 36
Association of Canadian Television and Radio Artists (ACTRA), 166
Avon Theatre, 154

B

Bacall, Lauren
  dialect usage of, 31, 37
back awareness, 53
back support difficulty
  explorations for, 128
Bancroft, Anne
  dialect usage of, 37
  use of mouth resonator, 91
Banff Center for the Arts, 23
Baroody, Margaret, 142
Barstow, Marjorie, 48, 52
Bassett, Angela
  healthy voice usage of, 7
Bates, Alan
  healthy voice usage of, 7
Bates, Kathy
  healthy voice usage of, 7
Bedford, Brian, 146
  warm-ups, 138
Beltran, Kyle, 108
Bening, Annette
  healthy voice usage of, 7
Benison, Ben, 118
Benjamin, Nancy, 39
Bennett, Fran, 16
Bentley, Kenajuan, 182
Berger, Zach, 28
Berkery, Barbara, 184
  dialect coaching by, 142
Bernardy, Danny, 180
Berry, Cicely, 14, 15, 19, 26, 40, 43, 111, 113, 115, 135, 138, 139, 182, 185
Berry method, 21, 24, 62, 112
  diversion tactics, 113, 182
  in group work, 182
  integration of voice and text in, 42
  text analysis in, 40
  text exercises, 71
  warm-up, 138

Big Day, 108
bioenergetics, 19
Birmingham Conservatory for
    Classical Theatre, 128
Black Book, 8
Blanchett, Cate
    healthy voice usage of, 7
blurring thoughts
    explorations for, 121
Blythe, Domini, 114
body mapping, 52
    in period costumes, 53
Bomer, Matthew, 85
Bonham Carter, Helena
    healthy voice usage of, 7
Boxer, The, 7
Boyfriend, The, 151, 174
Boyle, Lara Flynn
    unhealthy voice usage of, 9
Brando, Marlon
    dialect issues of, 144
breath support, 4, 5, 10, 15, 45
    accents/dialects, 145
    Alexander Technique, 46
    alignment, 45
    blocking scenes, 51
    with corset, 161
    exercises for, 13
    explorations for, 128
    healthy voice usage, 2
    lack of, 3, 46
    Linklater method, 17
    maintaining, 3, 4
    philosophies regarding, 20
    rib reserve, 20
    tongue twisters, 82
    writing exercises, 27
breathing
    control of, 227
    during speech, 225
    factors affecting, 226
    nasal, 224
        character choice for, 224

oral, 224
physiology of, 218
sounds during, 226
techniques for, 223
breathy voice, 3, 10, 32, 48, 67,
    229, 230
Bristol Old Vic, 43, 63, 71, 128
British actors
    and text analysis, 19
British dialect
    warm-ups, 146
British methods
    of voice/speech training, 42
broad phonetics, 35
Bryan, Kersti, 107
Bryne, Barbara, 103
Bullets over Broadway, 7
Bunch, Barbara, 19

C

California Institute of the Arts, 16,
    19
Campbell, Benedict, 140
Campbell, Brittany, 28
Campbell, Suzy Q., 157
Campion, Joyce
    injury and recovery of, 166
Canadian Actors' Equity (CAE), 166
Canadian Opera Company, 142
Canadian Stage, 166
Carnegie Mellon University, 4, 19,
    20, 21, 22, 24, 26, 27, 31,
    36, 37, 40, 46, 58, 85, 88,
    107, 108, 138, 152
Carrière, Bert, 174
Carrington, Walter, 48, 55
    support of actors, 51, 177
Cashmere Mafia, 108
Casino, 103
Catch Me If You Can, 7
Central School of Speech and
    Drama, 16, 19, 42, 43

Chaikin, Joe, 16
chair work
   in Alexander Technique, 56
character choices, vocal
      considerations for, 230
Charles, Gaius, 27, 85
Chasing Amy, 9
Chekhov, Anton
   plays of, 45, 50, 135, 183, 184
Cherry Orchard, The, 50
chest resonator, 90
   example of, 108
chest/back resonator, 92
   example of, 107
   Shakespearean text for, 94
   text for, 93
child actors
   feedback from vocal coach, 159
   issues with, 158
   time constraints of, 159
Christie, Julie
   healthy voice usage of, 7
Churchill, Caryl
   corset use, 161
Cider House Rules, 8
Cimolino, Antoni, 43, 155
Close, Glenn
   unhealthy voice usage of, 9
coaches
   appreciation of, 188
   compensation for, 166
   multiple
      and coordination of, 178
   support of actors and directors, 179
   timing of contribution, 172
Colaianni, Louis, 42
   about, 41
Colaianni method, 38
Columbia University, 17, 19, 35
Comedia exercise, 127
communication
   between coach and director, 183, 184
   between coaches, 185
Company of Women, The, 17
Conable, Barbara, 52
Conable, William, 52
confidentiality, respect for actors', 177
conscious control, 57
constructive rest
   in Alexander Technique, 54
contradictions between coach and director, 178
cool-down(s), 239
Cooper, Alec, 153
corset use
   actor's comfort, 157
   breath support, 156
   Vox Explora for, 161
   warm-ups for, 157
Corvin, Maria, 79
coughing
   harm of, 231
counseling, 24
Courage Under Fire, 9
Coward, Noel, 92
Cronyn, Hume
   preparation methods of, 169
Cruise, Tom
   healthy voice usage of, 7
   unhealthy voice usage of, 9
Crystal, Billy
   healthy voice usage of, 7
CSI Miami, 108
Cyrano de Bergerac
   voice strain in, 89

D

Daggett, Windsor P., 36
Das Leben der Anderen, 7, 8
Davis, Bette
   dialect usage of, 31
Davis, Carole
   use of Ybuzz resonator, 98

Day-Lewis, Daniel
  American dialect of, 143
  flawless dialect of, 147
  healthy voice usage of, 7
De Niro, Robert
  healthy voice usage of, 7
Depardieu, Gérard
  French accent of, 143
DePaul University, 41
descriptive approach(es)
  in speech training, 41
destructuring process, 19, 20
developing contrast
  explorations for, 122
dialect coaches, 142
dialect director, 165
dialect(s)
  breath support, 145
  British, 32
  coaches, 165
  coaching, 142, 145
  defined, 142
  denoting with symbols, 143
  early study of, 146
  interfering with performance, 144
  Irish, 145
  issues with learning, 145
  mid-Atlantic, 31, 32, 37
diaphragm, *218*
DiCaprio, Leonardo
  healthy voice usage of, 7
  unhealthy voice usage of, 9
director
  Alexander Technique training, 54
  and expectations of coach, 183
  pre-opening nerves of, 181
  and support of coach to actors, 183
distinguishing images
  explorations for, 122
diversion strategy, 113
  in Berry method, 182
Dracula, 8

dropping final words
  explorations for, 119
dropping in exercise, 114
dust in theater, 150

E

elisions, 36, 38
  avoiding in British dialect, 146
Emerson College, 17
emotion
  and the voice, 23
  in voice training, 25
emotional response
  actor's, 24
end gaining, 47
Entourage, 108
ENTs, 142
epithelium
  damage to, 216
equity breaks, 141
equity contracts for voice coaches, 166
Equus, 144
Eugene Grabscheid Voice Center, 142
excitation, 18
exhalation
  control of, 227
  described, 219
explorations for rehearsals, 57
extended voice approach (Roy Hart), 22

F

Farrow, Mia
  use of sinus resonator, 99
Feldenkrais method, 56, 161
  and Alexander Technique, 56
  and The Journey (Parks), 22
Feldenkrais, Moishe, 161
Fergus, Dylan, 85
Fertman, Bruce, 49, 50, 52

Fertman, Martha, 49, 50
fight choreography
   Alexander coach, 187
   Alexander Technique, 54
Firm, The, 7, 8
Fitzmaurice, Catherine, 19, 21
Fitzmaurice method, 19, 21, 29, 44, 62
   at Carnegie Mellon, 25
   destructuring process, 19
   exercises for corset use, 162
   inhibition in, 20
   philosophy of, 20
   singing, 28
   teachers of, 42
   voice support, 20
   voice work, 19
   warm-up, 138
   yoga in, 19
fog (special effect)
   and voice health, 149
Folkwang Hochschule, 54
Francis, Lynette, 63
Frederick, Michael
   and support of actors, 177
Freeman, Morgan
   healthy voice usage of, 8
French
   accents and dialects, 143
Friday Night Lights, 85
Fry, Ed
   use of Ybuzz resonator, 98

G

Gad, Joshua, 108
Galvin, Emma, 28
Gandolfini, James
   use of nasal resonator, 102
Garrard, Steffie, 28
Gedeck, Martha
   healthy voice usage of, 7
General American dialect, 31, 40
   inflections in, 143

Ybuzz resonator, 98
George Brown College, 79
Gepner-Mueller, Zoana, 65
getting across the argument
   explorations for, 124
Gilligan, Carol, 17
Glengarry Glen Ross, 8
Gods and Monsters, 8
Goldberg, Natalie, 26
good American speech, 36, 37, 41, 42
Good American stage speech, 31
   in Skinner method, 36
Goode, Kellie, 28
Gosford Park, 7, 8, 91, 102
Gould Center for the Care of the Voice, 142
Graduate, The, 37, 91
Greek texts, 27, 88
Green Card, 143
Greer, Germaine
   speeches of, 33
Griffin, Matthew, 108
Gross, Demetrius, 107
group work, 182
Guiding Light, 85
Guthrie Theater, 19, 43
Guzman, Paloma, 25

H

Hahn, Allen, 153
Haley, Robert, 39, 53
Hall, Albert
   use of mouth resonator, 91
Hamlet, 7, 9
   voice and text explorations in, 123
Hands, Brian, 142
hard palate
   defined, 4
Harris, Ed
   healthy voice usage of, 8
Harrow, Lisa, 38, 176

INDEX

Hart, Jonathan, 23
Hart, Roy, 22, 23
Hartley, Mary, 174
Hawkshaw, Mary, 142
Hawley, Alana, 128
head resonator
   defined, 103
   example of, 108
   guidelines for, 104
   with half masks, 158
   uses of, 104
Healey, Desmond, 53
Hecht, Deborah, 39
Henry IV
   voice and text explorations in, 123
Henry V, 8
Henry, Martha, 114, 128
   costume impact, 160
   warm-ups, 138
Hepburn, Katherine
   dialect usage of, 31
herbal treatments, 141
Hersan, Rita, 142
Herskovits, David, 138
Horowitz, Jeffrey, 43, 139, 155
Houseman, John, 36
Hunter, Holly, 33
hydration
   importance of, 141, 236
   and working out, 236
hyperadduction
   affects of, 232
hypoadduction
   affects of, 232

I

Ideal Husband, An, 7
Importance of Being Earnest, The, 188
In a Different Voice, 17
In the Name of the Father, 147
inhalation, described, 218
inhibition, 47

International Phonetic Alphabet, 14, 35, 42, 173
International Phonetics Association, 35
Interview with the Vampire, 9
Irish dialect, 143, 145
ischia, defined, 163

J

Jackson, Samuel L.
   healthy voice usage of, 8
Jenney, Alison
   healthy voice usage of, 7
Jernigan, David, 49
Jew of Malta, The, 121, 138, 171, 182, 185
Journey, The (Parks), 22, 29
Juilliard, 19, 21, 36, 39, 54, 72

K

Kavan, Nadia, 59
Kent State University, 31, 144, 157
kinesense, defined, 69
kinesthetic approaches, 37
King Lear
   nasal resonator in, 102
   sinus resonator in, 99
King, Martin Luther, Jr.
   speeches of, 33, 67, 71
Kinghorn, Deborah, 22
Kiselov, Mladen, 183
   use of diversion tactics, 182
Klick, Richard, 31
Kline, Kevin, 36
Knight, Dudley, 16, 42, 167
Knight method, 42
Koch, Sebastian
   healthy voice usage of, 8
Korovin, Gwen, 142
Krausnick, Dennis, 114, 115
Kron, Lisa, 26

L

Lada, Oksana
  use of Ybuzz resonator, 98
ladder of the thoughts, 125
  defined, 18
Lake, Ian, 129
Langford, Elizabeth, 55
Langham, Michael, 39
laryngeal cancer, 141
laryngologists, 140
larynx, 212
  extrinsic muscles of, 214
  hard structures of, 212
  hard tissue of, *213*
  intrinsic muscles of, 215, *216*
  musculature of, 214
  relation to head and neck, *212*
Lehane, Nick, 28
Lessac, Arthur, 21
Lessac method, 21, 29
  Lessac Kinesensic Training, 21
  Vox Explora warm-up, 76
  Ybuzz, 97
Lessac Training and Research Institute, 22
Lewis, Shelby, 28
lighting equipment
  ambient sounds of, 153
  description of, 153
  noise of fans, 154
Lincoln Center, 19
Lindo, Delroy
  healthy voice usage of, 8
Linklater Designation, 16, 41
Linklater exercises
  defined, 17
Linklater, Kristin, 16, 17, 24, 26, 87, 114, 115, 140
Linklater method, 16, 17, 18, 19, 20, 21, 29, 31, 44, 62, 88, 89, 119
  chest resonator in, 90
  head resonator in, 103
  philosophy of, 20
  resonators, 87, *Also see* Chapter 6
  Vox Explora warm-up, 77
  warm-up, 138
Linquist, Paul, 27
Lives of Others, The, 7, 8
Love's Labor's Lost
  sinus resonator in, 101

M

Macbeth, 140, 166
Macdonald, Brian, 174
Malcolm X, 33
Malcolm X, 8, 91, 93
Mandela, Nelson
  inauguration speech of, 67, 70
Mansell, Lilene, 36
March, Barbara, 114
Mardi Gras, 108
mask
  full, 158
  half
    resonance issues with, 158
    warm-ups for, 158
mask area, 88
  defined, 14
  warm-up for, 81
mask resonance
  defined, 234
McCallion, Michael, 43
McDermott, Dylan
  healthy voice usage of, 8
McKay, Tony, 108
McKellen, Ian
  and ensemble warm-ups, 66
  healthy voice usage of, 8
  in warm-ups, 139
McLean, Margaret Prendergast, 35, 36
means whereby, 47
Measure for Measure

teeth resonator in, 97
Medea, 38, 176
medications, 141
meditation
  in Vox Explora, 62
meetings, prerehearsal
  for director and coach, 167
Melton, Joan, 28
Merchant of Venice, The, 34, 138, 171, 182, 185
microphones
  adjusting sounds for, 152
  clarity with, 152
  foot, 153
  headpiece, 153
Midsummer Night's Dream, A, 43, 94, 178
  mouth resonator in, 91
  nasal resonator in, 102
  Ybuzz resonator in, 98
Mighty Aphrodite, 104
Miller, Carol, 156
Mirodan, Vladimir, 184
Mirren, Helen
  healthy voice usage of, 7
Mixon, Laura, 108
Monette, Richard, 43, 184
  warm-ups, 138
Monich, Timothy, 36, 144, 146
Monomania, 26, 27
monotone speech
  explorations for, 120
  lack of breath support, 46
  Resonex exercises for, 107
  unhealthy voice usage, 3
Moosa, Corey, 27
Mostly Martha, 7
moustache
  and text clarity, 157
mouth resonator, 4, 81, 90, 96
  example of, 107, 108
  uses of, 90, 101
Mühe, Ulrich

  healthy voice usage of, 8

N

Name of the Father, The, 7
Nappo, Vince, 182
nasal resonator, 4
  described, 101
  example of, 107
  qualities of, 102
  for "strange" vocal quality, 89
Nellis, Tom, 139
nervous system
  warming up, 66
New York University, 16, 36, 39, 54
Nicholson, Jack
  nasality of, 34
  use of nasal resonator, 102, 108
nodules, 141
Northam, Jeremy
  healthy voice usage of, 8
  use of teeth resonator, 96
notes
  for musical theater performers, 175
  from voice coach, 172
    framing of, 175
    timing of, 172
NPR's *Fresh Air*, 177
NUMB3RS, 108

O

O'Casey, Sean, 145
Odom, Leslie, 108
off voice, 10, 32
Oldman, Gary
  controversial voice usage of, 8
Olivier, Laurence
  healthy voice usage of, 8
  nasal and teeth resonator, 103
Open Theatre, 16

Oregon Shakespeare Festival, 108
Original Resonex, 27
Othello
   head resonator in, 104
   nasal resonator in, 103
otolaryngologist, 142
Ottiwell, Frank, 58

P

Pacino, Al
   healthy voice usage of, 8
Packer, Tina, 16, 114, 115
pain, in voice production, 240
Palmer method, 31, 88
Palmer, Robert, 88
Palminteri, Chazz
   controversial voice usage of, 8
Paltrow, Gwyneth
   and Standard British dialect, 142
Papp, Joseph, 32
Pappas, Ted, 38, 176
Parks method, 29
Parks, Robert, 22, 37, 58
Particular Class of Women, A, 49
Passy, Paul, 35
Pennell, Richard
   warm-ups, 138
Pesci, Joe
   use of snasal resonator, 103
Philadelphia Area Rep Theatre, 40
Phillips, Robin, 43
   use of diversion tactics, 114
   warm-ups, 138
phonation
   defined, 215, 220
   effects on, 234
   issues, 229
   physiology of, 220
   steam inhalers, 225
   vocal fold injury, 231
phonotrauma, 229

physiology
   of breathing, 218
   phonatory, 220
physiology of voice. *See* Appendix
pillows, phonetic symbol, 41
Pino, Joe, 152
pitch
   increase in, 215
Pitt, Brad
   healthy voice usage of, 8
   unhealthy voice usage of, 9
Pittsburgh Public Theater, 21, 38, 176
Place Des Arts in Montreal, 144
playing intention
   definition of, 111
Point Park University, 38, 39
polyps, 141
position of mechanical advantage, or "monkey" work, 56
Practice, The, 8, 9
praying to the gods
   in chest/back resonator, 96
prescriptive approach(es)
   in speech training, 35
Present Laughter, 92
pressed voice, 229, 233
Priest, 8
Primary Colors, 7
program billing for coaches, 165
Proval, David
   use of snasal resonator, 103
psychologists, 140
psychophysical approaches, 38
psychophysical aspects
   of Linklater method, 18
psychophysical voice work, 23, 28
Public Broadcasting Service, 43
Pulp Fiction, 8
pushed voice, 10
pushing vocally
   explorations for, 118

INDEX

Q
Queen, The, 7

R
r coloring, 37, 40
Raphael, Bonnie, 22
rapping
  in text exploration, 118
Received Pronunciation, 14, 36
reflux, 28, 141, 236
  described, 236
Resnick, Zak, 28
resonators
  exploring different, 106
  guidelines for using, 90
Resonex, 4, 87, *See* Chapter 6
  integrating into explorations, 106
  in rehearsals, 105
  with writing exercise, 107
respiratory muscles
  and loudness regulation, 228
Restoration play, 67
Restoration text
  use with teeth resonator, 96
restructuring process, 19
  defined, 20
Return to Love, 67
rhythm, lack of
  explorations for, 118
rib reserve, 20
Ribisi, Giovanni
  unhealthy voice usage of, 9
Richard III, 7, 8, 45, 114
  employing various resonators in, 105
  nasal resonator in, 103
Rickman, Alan, 177
Rifkin, Ron, 9
River Runs Through It, A, 8
Roache, Liam
  healthy voice usage of, 8
Rodenburg method
  warm-up, 138
Rodenburg, Patsy, 43, 71, 115, 118, 126
Rogal, Katie, 27
Romeo and Juliet, 9
Rosemary's Baby
  sinus resonator in, 99
Rosen, Clark, 142
Rousselot, Kylee, 27
Roy Hart Company, 23
Roy Hart method, 23, 28, 29
  development of, 22
  nasal resonator, 102
  resonating approaches of, 89
Roy Hart Theatre, 89
Royal Academy of Dramatic Art, 31, 118
Royal Alexandra Theatre, 142
Royal National Theatre, 44
Royal Shakespeare Company, 14, 40, 42, 43, 66, 111
  warm-ups, 139
Royal Shakespeare's Complete Works Festival, 139
rushing text
  explorations for, 115
Ryan, Meg
  unhealthy voice usage of, 9

S
Saks, Ethan, 28
salary negotiation for coaches, 165
Sataloff, Robert, 68, 140, 142
Scarface, 7
Scott Thomas, Kristin
  healthy voice usage of, 7
  use of mouth resonator, 91
screaming, training in, 231
screaming and yelling
  affects on voice, 230

Screen Actors Guild (SAG), 166
sense explorations, 129
Sex and the City, 98
Shadow of a Gunman, 145
Shakespeare, dialect in, 32
Shakespeare & Company, 16, 17, 24, 41, 114, 115, 116
Shakespeare in Love, 142
Shakespearean text
   head resonator in, 104
   nasal resonator in, 102
   practicing, 27
   sense explorations in, 131
   Ybuzz resonator in, 98
Shaw Festival, 63, 68
Shaw, George Bernard
   plays of, 67, 144
   practicing texts of, 27
Shawshank Redemption, The, 8
Shepard, Sam, 16
Sherman, Ashley, 27
Shoaf, Brian, 27
Shurtleff, Michael, 135, 136
singing (Fitzmaurice method), 28
singing teachers, 68, 140, 142
sinus resonator, 24, 81, 87
   example of, 108
   uses of, 99
Skinner, Edith, 22, 33, 35, 36, 37
Skinner method, 31, 36, 37, 38, 39, 40, 41, 88
   concerns with, 37
   good American stage speech in, 36
   problems with, 38
   rigidity of, 39
sleep, importance of, 240
Sling Blade, 8
small interpretation
   explorations for, 116
Smith, Liz, 72
Smith, Maggie
   nasality of, 34
   use of nasal resonator, 102
   warm-ups, 138
smoke (special effect), and voice health, 149
Smukler, David, 16, 31, 62, 115, 183
Smukler method
   warm-up, 138
snasal resonator, 82
   definition of, 103
   example of, 108
   for "tough guys", 103
Sopranos, The, 98, 103
Sorvino, Mira
   use of head resonator, 104
   use of nasal resonator, 104
sound and lighting cues
   during warm-ups, 66
sound cues, 150
   obscuring lines, 150
speaking voice training
   defined, 14
special effects
   guidelines for use, 149
   and voice health, 149
speech pathologists, 142
speech training
   defined, 14
   descriptive approaches to, 41
   prescriptive approaches to, 35
Spelling Bee, 108
Spin-a-Story, 129
spontaneity, developing
   explorations for, 126
squeezed or pushed voice, 10
stage whisper, 230
Standard British dialect, 14, 142, 145
   inflections in, 143
State University of New York (SUNY), 22
Stitt, Milan, 26

Stratford Shakespeare Festival, 4, 39, 40, 43, 53, 89, 103, 114, 128, 129, 140, 142, 151, 153, 154, 155, 156, 166, 170, 174
   warm-ups, 138
Streetcar Named Desire, A, 113, 135, 152
Stuart, Barbara, 114
suggestions, time for actors to process, 178
support of vocal coach, 176
swallowing text
   explorations for, 128
Sweet Briar Residential Alexander Summer Program, 49

T

table work in Alexander technique, 56
tai chi, and The Journey (Parks), 22
taking ownership
   explorations for, 117
Tandy, Jessica
   preparation methods of, 169
teeth resonator, 81, 89, 96
   description of, 96
   example of, 107
   Shakespearean text with, 96
Tempest, The, 151
Terms of Endearment, 102
text analysis
   by American actors, 19
   Berry method of, 40
   by British actors, 19
   healthy voice usage and, 133
   importance of, 133
   Resonex in, 105, 109
   sloppy, 5
   and vocal health, 61

text explorations, 115
text support
   explorations for, 129
theaters
   environmental irritants in, 237
Theatre for a New Audience, 43, 138, 155, 171, 185
   warm-ups at, 139
theatre space, adjusting to
   explorations for, 126
theme development difficulty
   explorations for, 125
Thomas, Francis, 43, 71, 115, 127, 128
Thompson, Emma
   healthy voice usage of, 7
Thompson, Phil, 42, 167
Thornton, Billy Bob
   controversial voice usage of, 8
thought difficulty
   explorations for, 125
Three Sisters, 134, 135, 183, 184
throat clearing
   harm of, 231
thyroid cartilage, 213
tight jaw
   explorations for, 119
Tilly, William, 35, 36
Tisch School of the Arts, 39
tongue twisters, 77
   examples, 83
   exercises, 39, 67, 75, 82
tonus, 48
tracheal pull, 225
Treco, Mathenee, 28
tremor, 20
Tresnjak, Darko, 138
Tru Calling, 85
Truth, Sojourner, 33, 67
Tukur, Ulrich
   healthy voice usage of, 8
Turner, Clifford, 19

tutorials
  on call sheet, 170
  one-on-one, 169
    elements of, 171
    length of, 170
    respect for, 170
    space for, 170
Twelfth Night
  head resonator in, 104
  mouth resonator in, 91
  sense explorations in, 130
  sinus resonator in, 100
  teeth resonator in, 96
  Ybuzz resonator in, 98

U

UCLA, 19, 27, 38, 40, 54
Uncle Vanya, 45, 134
unclear enunciation
  explorations for, 125
unintelligible speech
  explorations for, 124
University of California, Irvine, 16, 21, 42
University of Delaware, 19, 21
University of Kansas, 41
University of Pittsburgh, 142
University of the Arts theater program, 40
up and over the shelf, 5

V

Verdolini, Katherine, 142
vibratory cycle, *221*
Vickers, John, 68
Vickers William, 68
Vietor, Marc, 182
vocal cool-down, 5, 68
  elements of, 69
vocal exercises, 13
vocal fatigue, 140

vocal fold, *217*
  described, 216
  injury, 231
vocal function
  factors affecting, 222
vocal health, 139
  basic tips, 141
vocal hyperfunction
  signs of, 232
  types of, 232
vocal injuries, 140
vocal warm-up
  elements of, 66
  importance of, 66
vocal/dialect requirements
  coordination of, 167
voice
  acoustics issues, 234
  anatomy and physiology of. *See* Appendix
  breathy, 229
  conservation of, 238
  cool-downs, 239
  effects on, 234
  emotion, 23
  environmental factors affecting, 236
  hormonal influences on, 234
  hyperfunctional, 229
  hypofunctional, 229
  loudness
    increasing, 232
  pressed, 229
  production. *See* phonation and pain, 240
    technical parameters affecting, 223
  projection, 233
  quality of, 229
  rest of, 239
  screaming and yelling, 230
  use and rest, 237
  warm-up, 238

writing, 26
voice and speech study
   for directors, 67
Voice and Speech Trainers
   Association (VASTA), 42,
   143, 167
voice coach
  child actor issues, 159
  introduction of to cast, 168
  meetings with director, 168
voice training
  defined, 13
  goals of, 27
voice usage
  analysis checklist, 5
  controversial, 4
    examples, 8
  healthy, 2
    breath support in, 2
    examples, 7
    mechanics of, 136
  poor, 2, 3
  unhealthy
    breath support in, 3
    examples, 8
voice/dialect coaches
  salary and billing, 165
voice/text director, 165
voice-in-the-mouth resonator
  use of, 92
voicing, described, 222
Volsen, Alfred, 22
Vox Cura, 142
Vox Explora. *See* all of Chapter 5
  daily warm-ups, 138
  definition of, 62
  floor exercises, 77
  Resonating Ladder exercises,
    80
  standing exercises, 79
  warm-up
    lying down, 72
    standing, 71

W

Wade, Andrew, 43, 112, 113, 115
Wade method
  warm-up, 138
Wadsworth, Don, 40
Wagar method, 38
  text analysis in, 40
Wagar, Paul, 40
Waiting to Exhale, 7
Walsh, Robin, 39
warm-up(s)
  for British dialect, 146
  for corset use, 161
  director's support of, 138
  elements of, 68
  established actors, 138
  importance of, 137
  length of, 138
  scheduling, 138
Warren, Iris, 16, 79
Washington, Denzel, 93
  healthy voice usage of, 8
Weaver, Sigourney
  healthy voice usage of, 7
Webber Douglas Drama School, 40
Welles, Orson
  use of mid-Atlantic dialect, 37
West Wing, The, 7
whisper
  "easy", 230
whispering, 230
  harm of, 230
  when hoarse, 141
Wiest, Dianne
  healthy voice usage of, 7
Williams, David, 43
Williams, Tennessee
  plays of, 113, 135
    dialects in, 147
Williamson, Marianne, 67
Wings of the Dove, 7
Winslow Boy, The, 8, 96

Woo, Peak, 142
Working Girl, 7
working out
   and hydration, 236
Working Theatre, 16
writing
   as a voice exercise, 26

Y

Yale University, 19, 21, 54
Ybuzz resonator
   about, 97
   example of, 107, 108
   uses of, 98
yoga, 19
   compared to voice work, 65
   in Fitzmaurice method, 19
York University, 16, 19, 62
Young Company, 188

Z

Zito, Ralph, 39